Prevention of Contact Dermatitis

Current Problems in Dermatology

Vol. 25

Series Editor *G. Burg,* Zurich

KARGER

Basel · Freiburg · Paris · London · New York · New Delhi · Bangkok · Singapore · Tokyo · Sydney

Prevention of Contact Dermatitis

Volume Editors *P. Elsner,* Zurich
J.M. Lachapelle, Brussels
J.E. Wahlberg, Stockholm
H.I. Maibach, San Francisco, Calif.

70 figures, 1 in color, and 52 tables, 1996

KARGER

Basel · Freiburg · Paris · London · New York ·
New Delhi · Bangkok · Singapore · Tokyo · Sydney

Current Problems in Dermatology

Library of Congress Cataloging-in-Publication Data
International Conference on the Prevention of Contact Dermatitis (1995: Zurich, Switzerland)
Prevention of contact dermatitis: the epidemiological basis / International Conference on the Prevention of Contact Dermatitis, Zurich, October 4–7, 1995; volume editors, P. Elsner ... [et al.].
(Current problems in dermatology; vol. 25)
Includes bibliographical references and index.
1. Contact dermatitis – Prevention – Congresses. 2. Contact dermatitis – Epidemiology – Congresses. I. Elsner, Peter, 1955– . II. Title. III. Series.
[DNLM: 1. Dermatitis, Contact – prevention & control – congresses. 2. Dermatitis, Contact – epidemiology – congresses. W1 CU804L v.25 1996 / WR 175 I61 1996]
RL244.I58 1995
616.97′305 – dc20
ISBN 3–8055–6311–6 (hardcover: alk. paper)

Bibliographic Indices. This publication is listed in bibliographic services, including Current Contents® and Index Medicus.

Drug Dosage. The authors and the publisher have exerted every effort to ensure that drug selection and dosage set forth in this text are in accord with current recommendations and practice at the time of publication. However, in view of ongoing research, changes in government regulations, and the constant flow of information relating to drug therapy and drug reactions, the reader is urged to check the package insert for each drug for any change in indications and dosage and for added warnings and precautions. This is particularly important when the recommended agent is a new and/or infrequently employed drug.

Printed in Switzerland on acid-free paper by Thür AG Offsetdruck, Pratteln
ISBN 3–8055–6311–6

Contents

Prevention of Irritant Contact Dermatitis

Prevention of Allergic Contact Dermatitis

Exposure Assessment and Risk Group Targeting in Contact Dermatitis Prevention

Secondary Prevention

Gloves

Protective Creams and Moisturizers

Preface

Contact dermatitis (CD) is an environmental disease par excellence: Without skin contact to irritants or allergens no one will develop CD. Furthermore, it is an extremely frequent, chronic and possibly disabling disease resulting in considerable economic damage to the individual and the community. Thirdly, it is basically a preventable disease, and prevention is a must considering that therapy is symptomatic and often of limited value.

While dermatologists do a marvellous job in diagnosing CD and elucidating its causes, CD prevention has been a neglected aspect of clinical dermatology. As a matter of fact, CD prevention is something that should not happen in hospitals or practices, but in the daily life of workers and consumers. Therefore, an integrated approach is needed involving many specialties: (1) chemists, toxicologists, pharmacists and cosmetologists in the risk prediction of chemicals and in the formulation of products; (2) safety engineers and occupational physicians in the assessment and minimization of risks at the workplace; (3) clinical dermatologists and allergologists in the early detection of new causes of CD and in secondary and tertiary prevention; (4) epidemiologists in the detection of target populations and situations for preventive action; (5) preventive medicine and public health specialists in the planning and realization of prevention projects; (6) economists and insurance specialists in the balancing of cost and benefit of preventive activities; (7) legislators in the definition of the legal requirements and regulating agencies in their application to the real world.

Valuable knowledge on disease prevention exists in all of the mentioned specialties, but this is the first time this information has been brought together in a text devoted to the preventive aspects of CD. We hope that this book will be useful both for planning preventive strategies and for the prevention of CD in the daily practice of dermatologists and occupational physicians.

The editors would like to thank the contributors, all experts in the field, for their precise work and harmonious cooperation. Ms. Vogelhuber, Department of Dermatology, University of Zurich, provided important secretarial assistance. Without the kind support by the publisher, Dr. h.c. Thomas Karger, his technical staff, Ms. Liza Anyawike and Susanna Ludwig, and without the encouragement of the series editor, Prof. G. Burg, the making of this book would not have been possible.

Peter Elsner, MD, Zurich
Jean-Marie Lachapelle, MD, Brussels
Jan Wahlberg, MD, Stockholm
Howard I. Maibach, MD, San Francisco

Elsner P, Lachapelle JM, Wahlberg JE, Maibach HI (eds): Prevention of Contact Dermatitis. Curr Probl Dermatol. Basel, Karger, 1996, vol 25, pp 1–9

Epidemiological Studies on the Prevention of Occupational Contact Dermatitis

Thomas L. Diepgen

Department of Dermatology (Chairman: Prof. Dr. *G. Schuler*), Friedrich-Alexander University Erlangen-Nuremberg, Germany

The ideal role of a medical practitioner involved in occupational dermatology is not only to diagnose and treat patients, but also to determine the etiology of the occupational skin disease and to make recommendations for its prevention. In this paper I would like to demonstrate that understanding the epidemiology of occupational contact dermatitis (OCD), that is, knowing the distribution and determinants of disease frequencies, can assist in accomplishing these tasks. OCD is a preventable disease and only through the knowledge of its epidemiological characteristics can the goal of prevention be achieved.

Epidemiological studies can be categorized as descriptive, etiologic, and intervention studies. Descriptive studies demonstrate the public health importance, characterize the demographics of the affected population, and identify hazards and risks. Etiologic studies examine risk factors, prognostic factors, and the natural history of OCD. Intervention studies evaluate the effectiveness of measures to prevent or reduce the impact of OCD.

The information from these studies may provide answers to the following clinically important questions: (1) What is the public health importance and impact of OCD? (2) How large are prevalence and incidence? (3) What industries are associated with a higher risk for workers? (4) What are the occupational exposures causing OCD? (5) Who is at risk? (6) What is the prognosis of patients with OCD? (7) What preventive measures and interventions are effective?

Public Health Importance and Impact of OCD

Occupational skin diseases account for 30–40% of all cases of occupational illness in industrial countries [1, 2]. The incidence rate of registered occupational skin diseases in most countries lies at around 0.5–0.7 cases per 1,000 full-time workers per year [1]. Contact dermatitis localized mostly at the hands accounts for the vast majority of work-related dermatoses [2, 3]. The economic impact of OCD can be measured using clinical, economic and social measures and is very high according to the following costs: (a) direct cost of medical care, workers' compensation or disability payments; (b) indirect costs associated with lost workdays and loss of productivity; (c) costs of occupational retraining; (d) costs attributable to the effects on the quality of life.

The total annual costs of OCD might have ranged from USD 222 million to 1 billion in the US 10 years ago [3]. These estimates do not include costs of occupational retraining which accounts for about DM 100,000–200,000 per case in Germany. There are no recent studies on the costs attributable to the effects on the quality of life.

Prevalence and Incidence of OCD in Different Industries

One of the most basic questions is the frequency with which occupational contact dermatitis and sensitizations against various allergens occur [4]. The availability of such data is a prerequisite for any systematic investigation of patterns of disease occurrence in human populations. Studies among patient populations from dermatology clinics are not adequate for estimating prevalence or incidence rates. All measures of disease frequency consist of the number of cases in the numerator, and the size of the population under study in the denominator. Among patient populations, however, the sample of the numerator is very often biased and the size of the denominator unknown. According to some population-based studies the frequency of hand eczema ranges between 2 and 10% [4]. How can the estimated incidence of occupational hand eczema be 100-fold smaller? Because of methodological aspects, like the definition of the outcome variable, differences in the study population, the study design, the used instruments, and the difficulties of systematic errors the published data are not comparable (table 1). There are several reasons that we only see the tip of the iceberg of occupational contact dermatitis. One of the most important problems is the lack of a standard case definition. Data sources may be based on employer reporting, employee self-reporting, patch test results, worker's compensation claims, and clinical diagnosis. This leads

Table 1. Methodological aspects of epidemiological studies on occupational contact dermatitis

Measures of frequencies	prevalence (point, period) cumulative incidence, incidence rate
Case ascertainment	instruments (questionnaire, dermatological examination) outcome variable (self-reported, medical consultation due to OCD, sick leave) severity (mild, moderate, severe)
Errors	random errors (variability, precision, misclassification) systematic errors (selection bias, information bias, confounding)
Risk assessment	cohort studies (relative risk, attributable risk percent) case-control studies (odds ratio)

to potential misclassification of OCD, resulting in overestimation or underestimation of disease frequency.

We are currently performing a prospective survey of all closed cases of OCD in North Bavaria [2]. In a 3-year period (3/1990 to 3/1993) in total 2,567 cases of work-related skin disease were stated. In cooperation with the German State Institute of Labour and Occupation the number of all employees of this referral area were evaluated for the same time period. Because all cases of OCD have been recorded and the number of employees during the same time period in the same referral area is known, incidence rates for a 3-year period could be calculated for different professions (fig. 1). The highest incidences were found in hairdressers, bakers, electroplaters, grinders, drillers and others. For the prevention of contact dermatitis it is important to know that mostly young employees develop OCD. The median of age in hairdressers, the food industry, health service, and metalworkers varied between 19 and 33 years. The induction period was very short: 2.1 years in hairdressers, 3.1 years in the food industry, 3.8 years in the health service, and 4.0 years in metalworkers.

Occupational Exposures Causing OCD

Identification of risk factors can result in a better understanding of the pathways leading to disease acquisition and thereby suggest preventive strategies. The development of occupational contact dermatitis is determined by a combination of exposure characteristics and individual susceptibility (fig. 2). Skin contact with irritants and allergens is a necessary condition, but the

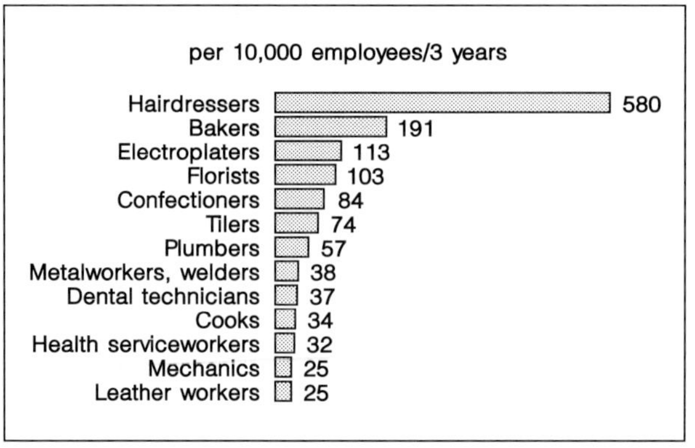

Fig. 1. Three-year incidence rates of occupational skin diseases in North Bavaria.

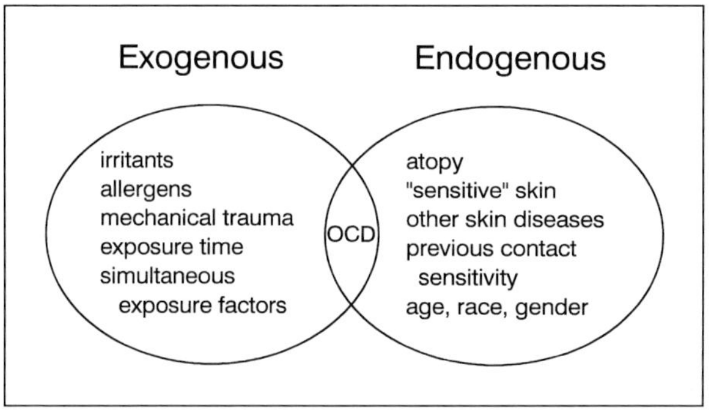

Fig. 2. The interrelationship between exogenous and endogenous risk factors for OCD.

probability and severity of a reaction depend on the type and intensity of exposure. Additionally, apart from exposure to hazardous substances there are many endogenous factors that may influence the development of OCD, such as atopic constitution, psychological factors, age, gender. Environmental factors may play a role in this process by influencing the individual susceptibility and the characteristics of exposure. If these factors are not properly controlled either in the design or in the analysis, they may act as confounders in the study.

The most important risk factor is the exposure to irritants. Out of 145 grouped exposure sources the 5 most frequently stated substances were detergents, water, metals, foodstuff and rubber in notified occupational skin diseases in Denmark [5]. These substances cause approximately half of the eczema

Table 2. Principles and range of prevention measures for occupational contact dermatitis

1	Elimination or replacement of harmful substances (irritants, allergens)
2	Technical measures (e.g. encapsulation of the process, automation)
3	Organization (e.g. wet work distributed to all employees)
4	Personal protection (e.g. gloves, barrier creams, after-work creams, soaps)
5	Preemployment screening

cases. The most important irritant seems to be wet work. The highest priority in the cascade of prevention measures are elimination or replacement of harmful exposures (table 2). Therefore, it is important to analyze the distribution of sensitizations in different professions. In hairdressers we know the work-related allergens very well. According to our study in North Bavaria we are able to demonstrate that glycerylmonothioglycolate (GMTG), *p*-phenylendiamin, ammonium persulfate and toluylendiaminsulfate are the most frequent sensitizers and the most frequent occupational relevant allergens. In contrast, sensitizations to nickel are frequent, but nickel very rarely plays an occupational relevant role in hairdressers. In contrast, most of the OCD are caused by irritants in metalworkers. It is difficult to identify occupational important allergens in this work force. Most of the sensitizations diagnosed in our North Bavarian study are caused by substances from the standard series. Quite few of these sensitizations are occupational relevant.

There are, however, limitations and problems of epidemiological studies examining the risk of sensitization agents. Exposure is characterized by concentration and duration. Without doubt, exposure is the most important determinant of risk, but exposure quantification techniques are underdeveloped in dermatology. Exposure change with time, and the affected worker may continue to have eczema yet no longer exposed to the causative agent. The evaluation of past exposure may be exceedingly difficult which leads to recall and information bias. Because of unique exposure the results of a study are not generalizable. Cross-sectional studies are subject to survivor bias because subjects with severe skin diseases often leave the work force (healthy worker effect).

Role of Endogenous Factors

A challenging question for epidemiologists and dermatologists to solve together is: Given the situation where occupational exposure occurs, why is it that some workers develop eczema and others do not? This type of question

Table 3. Relative risk and etiologic fraction for subjects with atopic skin diathesis (ASD) in bakers with notified occupational contact dermatitis (n = 107)

Assumed frequencies of ASD in the general population %	Relative risk (95% CI)	Etiologic fraction %
5	18.8 (13.0; 27.0)	51
10	9.7 (6.7; 14.1)	49
15	6.3 (4.4; 9.2)	46
20	4.6 (3.1; 6.6)	42

The frequency of ASD in diseased bakers was 61%. Modified according to Tacke et al. [7].

requires carefully designed prospective studies. The results will hopefully provide further clues on effective methods of protection and care for susceptible individuals in situations where exposure cannot be avoided or further reduced. The role of atopy in occupational skin diseases was examined by reviewing the files of all closed cases (n = 958) in South Carolina [6]. Only 134 patients (13.9%) responded. 82% of these subjects were atopics and the authors analyzed the data as follows: assuming a 25% frequency of atopy in the general population the relative odds of developing ASD are 13.5 times greater if one is atopic. It is obvious that this figure may be heavily influenced by selection bias.

In bakers, we could demonstrate that atopic skin diathesis is the most important endogenous risk factor [7]. Assuming different frequency figures of atopic skin diathesis in the general population the relative risk for atopic subjects to develop occupational contact dermatitis differs between 4.6 and 18.8 (table 3). The attributable risk or etiologic fraction represents the proportion of ASD that can be explained by the risk factor. The etiologic fraction was between 42 and 51%.

Prospective, incidence-type studies should have priority. In prospective cohort studies we investigate the risk to develop occupational hand eczema in hairdressers, nurses and metalworkers [8,9]. The design of the study comprises a first dermatological investigation at the start of the apprenticeship and thereafter regular follow-ups over a 3-year period. In the first year of apprenticeship 68% of the hairdressers developed mild, moderate or severe hand eczema. It is important to examine simultaneously occupational and domestic exposure, endogenous disposition and skin protection measures when analyzing risk factors of ASD. An important statistical problem is, however, that skin-care habits change with the occurrence of hand eczema. Subjects with hand eczema change their skin care habits more often than apprentices without skin problems. Apprentices with hand eczema use gloves more often than healthy apprentices. This leads to a methodological problem: If skin protection measures are associated with the outcome of variable hand eczemas, they cannot be incorporated in a multivariate analysis. Therefore, it would be more appropriate to perform an intervention study to learn more about the role of skin protection measures in the prevention of occupational contact dermatitis.

In a multivariate analysis the two most important endogenous factors, atopic skin diathesis and respiratory atopy, were simultaneously analyzed with the history of nickel sensitivity and the following exogenous factors: duration of wet work and duration of permanent wave, because GMTG is one of the most important allergens. Because of the above-mentioned methodological difficulties skin protection measures were not included in this analysis. By a logistic regression model it can be demonstrated that atopic skin diathesis, wet work (more than 4 h daily) and permanent wave (more than 1 h daily) are the most important independent risk factors. The odds ratios (OR) and the corresponding 95% confidence intervals were as follows: $OR_{\text{atopic skin diathesis}}$ 2.1 (1.4, 3.2), $OR_{\text{respiratory atopy}}$ 0.8 (0.4, 1.4), $OR_{\text{wet work}}$ 2.1 (1.4, 3.0), $OR_{\text{permanent wave}}$ 1.7 (1.1, 2.4). In contrast, a history of nickel sensitivity was not associated with a significantly elevated risk for hand eczema: $OR_{\text{history of nickel sensitivity}}$ 1.3 (0.9, 1.9). The logistic regression model assumes a multiplicative model, which means in our example that the risk is 7.5-fold elevated if all three risk factors are given.

It should be noted that atopic hand eczema in childhood seems to be the most important risk factor for hand eczema in adults [10]. This study also found, however, that a considerable number of subjects with a personal history of atopic eczema managed to work in risk occupations without developing HE. Therefore, a reduced resistance to work-related irritants and allergens does not occur in all subjects with atopic eczema and may occur in subjects with respiratory atopy and in nonatopics. Lammintausta [11] introduced the term atopic skin diathesis (ASD) as a prognostically useful definition of the skin condition which might be involved in the development of hand eczema. In order to establish a diagnostic score of ASD we evaluated the basic and minor features of atopic eczema systematically in established cases of atopic eczema and in subjects randomly collected from the Caucasian normal population of young adults in a prospective computerized study [12]. On the basis of statistical modelling a diagnostic score system was constructed, which should be based on anamnestic and clinical features without laboratory investigations [4, 12].

Table 4. Intervention-type epidemiological studies are needed to prove the effectiveness of prevention measures in the work environment

Industrial process
Substitute less irritating/sensitizing agents
Reduce skin contact
Appropriate protective gloves
Education
Workers and management
Reduce skin contact
Job procedures training
Recognition and treatment of skin disease
Skin care program
Choice of cleansers, barrier creams, after-work creams, protective clothing

Effectiveness of Preventive Measures and Interventions

Recurring symptoms in working populations varied between 35 and 80%. Healing of OCD may or may not be influenced by a change in occupation. Because patients with OCD notoriously have a poor prognosis for clearing their skin diseases, the primary prevention of OCD is most important. As mentioned in table 2, strategies in the prevention of occupational contact dermatitis include identifying allergens and irritants, substituting chemicals that are less irritating or allergenic, establishing engineering controls to reduce exposure, and organizing the work in a way that all employees are exposed at the same degree. Personal protection, for example gloves or using barrier cream, and selection of less susceptible individuals have to be the last measures. Epidemiological studies on the prevention of contact dermatitis in the work environment are needed (table 4). There is a lack of intervention studies which are needed to prove the effectiveness of preventive measures and interventions. For example, the addition of ferrous sulfate to cement seems to be beneficial to reduce the occurrence of allergic contact dermatitis in bricklayers. The prevalence of chromate allergy in cement workers had fallen from 11 to 3% in Denmark [13].

The use of personal protective equipment must be considered carefully because it may create skin problems by occlusion and irritation. The effectiveness of barrier creams is also controversial and there is a lack of epidemiological studies dealing with the beneficial effects of these measures. The misuse of soaps and detergents can directly provoke irritant contact dermatitis of the hands. Therefore, additional interventions are needed, which include providing advice on the proper use of gloves and barrier creams, and educating the work force about exposure and skin care. To learn more about the impact of these measures it would be important to perform prospective, intervention-type studies.

In conclusion, very few truly epidemiological studies have been published which were aimed at the aspects of prevention of occupational contact dermatitis. The results of the different types of epidemiological studies (descriptive, etiologic, and intervention studies) will give better information on the prevalence and incidence of OCD, endogenous and exogenous risk factors, etiologic agents, prognostic factors, and preventive measures. This knowledge will help the dermatologist to play a key role in the prevention of occupational contact dermatitis.

References

1 Coenraads PJ, Smit J: Epidemiology, in Rycroft RJG, Menné, T, Frosch PJ, Benezra C (eds): Textbook of Contact Dermatitis. Berlin, Springer, 1992, pp 133–149.

2 Diepgen TL, Schmidt A, Schmidt M, Fartasch M: Demographic and legal characteristics of occupational skin diseases. Allergologie 1994;17:84–89.

3 Mathias CGT: The cost of occupational skin disease. Arch Dermatol 1985;121:332–334.

4 Diepgen TL, Coenraads, PJ: What can we learn from epidemiological studies on irritant contact dermatitis; in Elsner P, Maibach HI (eds): Irritant Dermatitis: New Clinical and Experimental Aspects. Basel, Karger, 1995, vol 23, pp 18–27.

5 Halkier-Sorensen L, Thestrup-Pedersen K: Anmeldte og anerkendte arbejdsbetingede hudsygdomme i Danmark. Copenhagen, Industriens Forlag, 1994.

6 Keil JE, Shmunes E: The epidemiology of work-related skin diseases in South Carolina. Arch Dermatol 1983;119:650–654.

7 Tacke J, Schmidt A, Fartasch M, Diepgen TL: Occupational contact dermatitis in bakers, confectioners and cooks: A population-based study. Contact Dermatitis 1995;33:112–117.

8 Funke U, Diepgen TL, Fartasch M: Identification of high-risk groups for irritant contact dermatitis by occupational physicians; in Elsner P, Maibach HI (eds): Irritant Dermatitis: New Clinical and Experimental Aspects. Basel, Karger, 1995, vol 23, pp 64–72.

9 Diepgen TL, Tepe A, Pilz B, Schmidt A, Hüner A, Huber A, Hornstein OP, Frosch PJ, Fartasch M: Occupational skin diseases in hairdressers and nurses during apprenticeship: Design of a prospective epidemiological study. Allergologie 1993;10:396–403.

10 Rystedt I: Hand eczema and long-term prognosis in atopic dermatitis (thesis). Acta Derm Venereol (Stockh) 1985;117:1–59.

11 Lammintausta K, Kalimo K: Atopy and hand dermatitis in hospital wet work. Contact Dermatitis 1981;7:301–308.

12 Diepgen TL, Fartasch M: Recent epidemiological and genetic studies in atopic dermatitis. Acta Derm Venereol (Stockh) 1992;(suppl 176):13–18.

13 Avnstorp C: Prevalence of cement eczema in Denmark before and since addition of ferrous sulfate to Danish cement. Acta Derm Venereol (Stockh) 1989;69:151–155.

Priv.-Doz. Dr. Thomas L. Diepgen, Department of Dermatology, Dermato-Epidemiology Unit, Hartmannstrasse 14, D–91052 Erlangen (Germany)

Elsner P, Lachapelle JM, Wahlberg JE, Maibach HI (eds): Prevention of Contact Dermatitis. Curr Probl Dermatol. Basel, Karger, 1996, vol 25, pp 10–17

Relative and Attributable Risk and Its Relevance to the Prevention of Contact Dermatitis

Hywel C. Williams

Dermatoepidemiology Unit, Queen's Medical Center, University Hospital, Nottingham, UK

'A little bit of harm affecting a lot of people can add up to more than a lot of harm affecting a few people'

The Problem

When investigating a potential risk factor for contact dermatitis, most researchers are comfortable with the concept of relative risk as an indicator of strength of an association. Thus, it is entirely appropriate for a researcher, having found that exposure to a hypothetical subtance called 'zickel' is associated with a relative risk of 100 for developing contact dermatitis, to then claim that 'zickel is a potent sensitiser'. Problems begin, however, when researchers get carried away with the importance of their own work and proceed to declare to the world that 'zickel is an important cause of contact dermatitis'. Such a statement requires careful consideration of the health impact of that substance in *absolute* terms, as well as consideration of wider public health issues such as cost-effectiveness of prevention programmes, and the possible negative effects of abolishing that substance versus implementing alternative protective measures with respect to the population at risk.

This chapter highlights the difference between the two main measures of risk, namely relative risk and attributable risk, and discusses their relevance to the prevention of contact dermatitis using real and hypothetical examples. Devoting an entire chapter to this topic may seem extravagant, but the conceptual jump from investigating and treating individuals to consideration of the health needs of an entire population is one which many physicians find difficult.

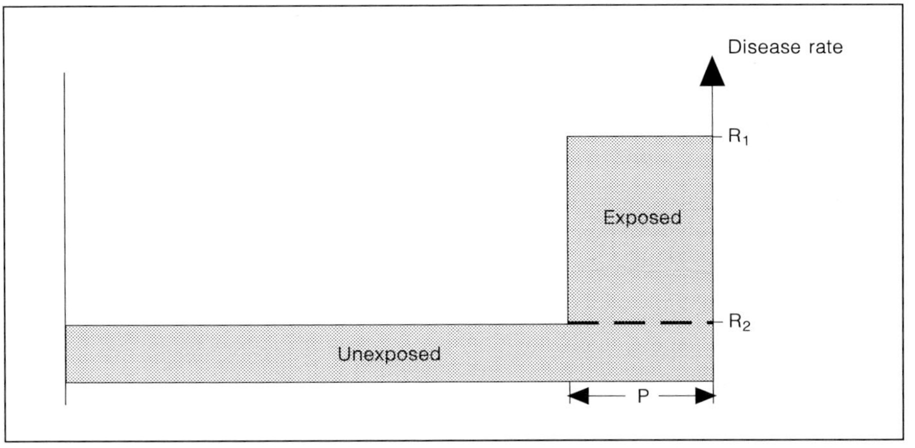

Fig. 1. Calculation of relative and attributable risk. P denotes the prevalence of exposure. Relative risk = rate in exposed/rate unexposed = R_1/R_2; attributable risk = (risk in exposed – rate unexposed) = $R_1 - R_2$.

It is inevitable that those engaged in contact dermatitis research will occasionally be required to advise authorities, and sometimes they will be involved in developing and executing prevention programmes themselves. It is important that all those interested in preventing contact dermatitis become familiar with some of the principles involved in assessing public health needs.

Some Theory

Relative Risk

Relative risk is a *ratio* measure. It may be defined as the ratio of the risk of disease in those exposed to a particular factor divided by the risk of disease in those who are not exposed, as shown in figure 1. Relative risk is often used as a measure of etiological strength for exploring possible risk factors for contact dermatitis such as atopic dermatitis or trauma.

In his lectures on the criteria for disease causality, Bradford-Hill [1] pointed out that very large relative risks are supportive of a causal link. Thus, given that the death rate for lung cancer in heavy cigarette smokers is 20–30 times as great as the rate in non-smokers, Bradford-Hill argued that it is unlikely that such a strong association could be explained by chance, bias or confounding. Interpretation of relative risk is straightforward when referring to an individual who asks the question 'How much more likely am I to develop lung cancer

Table 1. The paradox of relative and attributable risk in relation to deaths from smoking [4]

	Deaths from smoking	
	lung cancer	heart disease
Relative risk	14.0	1.6
Attributable risk	$130/10^5$/year	$256/10^5$/year

if I am a heavy smoker when compared with a non-smoker?' In simple terms, a relative risk of 30 indicates that a heavy smoker is 30 times more likely to develop lung cancer than a non-smoker. This does not necessarily mean that a heavy smoker will develop lung cancer (the author's grandfather smoked 30 cigarettes per day without any apparent harm), but that the *probability* of developing diseases is very much higher in such an individual [2]. A relative risk of one (1.0) implies no difference in risk, whereas a relative risk of less than one implies a possible protective effect. Relative risk measures are usually bounded by 95% confidence intervals to provide the reader with some indication of the precision of the estimate [3]. When the 95% confidence interval cross unity, the finding is not statistically significant at the 5% level. Thus, a relative risk of 4.2 (95%, 0.8–7.6) indicates a non-statistically significant increased relative risk, although it is possible that a larger sample could have yielded a statistically significant result.

Relative risk is not a good measure of public health impact since it is usually used to denote the probability of disease occurring in individuals as opposed to a particular population. It can be estimated in cohort and case-control studies [2].

Attributable Risk and Other Measures of Population Impact

Attributable risk is a *difference* measure. It may be defined as the difference between the incidence rate in the exposed and unexposed population as shown in figure 1. Attributable risk is a measure of the *absolute* effect of an exposure in a given population. Thus, in the example shown in table 1, the attributable risk for lung cancer due to smoking is 130 per 100,000 per year [4]. Attributable risk is an easier measure for those involved in planning health care for entire populations to interpret because it quantifies the excess risk associated with an exposure in absolute terms (NB, assuming that the association between exposure and disease is one of cause and effect). Attributable risk is usually only calculated from cohort studies. Although attributable risk refers to the absolute effect of exposure on an entire population, individuals may also be interested to know by how much their probability of disease will be reduced in real terms by choosing a particular preventive measure, e.g. reduction in cholesterol intake, weight loss, or exercise in relation to ischaemic heart disease.

Other measures of population impact derived from attributable risk are also used to assist in making public health decisions. *Population attributable* risk is a measure of the hypothetical effect that removal of an exposure would have on the rate of disease in the total population, and is calculated by multiplying the attributable risk by the prevalence of exposure. A more widely used and more easily understood measure is the *etiologic fraction* (population attributable risk fraction). Etiologic fraction denotes the percentage of disease incidence attributable to a particular exposure in a given population. It may be calculated by dividing the population attributable risk by the overall rate of disease in the population. Other formulae are sometimes used for estimating etiologic fraction from case control studies [2]. Thus, in relation to smoking and psoriasis, the author estimated that as much as one quarter of all disease could be attributed to smoking, if indeed a causal relationship existed [5]. Despite the usefulness of etiologic fraction in estimating the public health impact of various exposures, it is seldom seen in journals relating to contact dermatitis.

Some Examples

At this stage, it may seem obvious that the most appropriate measure for estimating the public health impact of a particular exposure is the attributable risk or one of its derivatives. Although exposures which confer a high relative risk of disease are accompanied by a high attributable risk in many circumstances, this is not always the case. Before scenarios in contact dermatitis are discussed, one classic example from general medicine deserves special mention – that of smoking-related deaths [4].

Sir Richard Doll and Deaths From Smoking

Table 1 illustrates relative and attributable risk of death from smoking broken down into deaths from lung cancer and deaths from heart disease. Given that relative risk of death from lung cancer due to smoking is far higher than that from heart disease (14.0 and 1.6, respectively), it may seem tempting to advise those implementing public health prevention programmes that the main impact of cessation of smoking will be on deaths from lung cancer. But inspection of attributable risks reveals a very different picture with nearly twice as many deaths from heart disease due to smoking when compared with lung cancer. This paradox can be explained by the fact that cardiovascular disease is a far more common disease than lung cancer, and a little bit of harm affecting a lot of people may add up to more than a lot of harm affecting a few people in absolute terms. Relative risk is therefore a poor predictor of attributable risk when viewed in isolation [2].

Closer to home, let us now consier some hypothetical examples of the clinical significance of each risk measure in relation to contact dermatitis.

Irritant Contact Dermatitis

In the example of deaths from smoking, we considered one exposure (smoking) and two disease outcomes (lung cancer and ischaemic heart disease). The situation is slightly different with irritant contact dermatitis (ICD), since we are dealing with one disease outcome – that is, the clinical picture which results in the diagnosis of ICD [6]. This next example demonstrates how prevalence of exposure must also be taken into account in assessing public health impact by measuring the etiologic fraction.

Consider a general population sample of 100,000 individuals where the overall rate of ICD is 2% (2,000/10^5/year), as shown in table 2. Although water-based cutting oils are associated with a far higher relative risk of developing ICD when compared with exposure to washing-up liquid, it accounts for only 8.0% of the total of ICD cases, compared with a staggering 37.5% from washing-up liquid. The mere fact that so many people are exposed to washing-up liquid makes this a more important factor in public health terms because it accounts for a greater proportion of the total disease burden. Of course, the situation may be different if the reference population were metal workers where cutting oils were used frequently [7], but even in this situation, it is often surprising how much ICD can be due to frequent hand washing using harsh cleansers, rather than contact with water-based cutting oils. Any intervention in such a situation requires an evaluation of the attributable risk and prevalence of exposure.

Allergic Contact Dermatitis (ACD)

Suppose that two previous separate publications had shown that the relative risk for the clinical picture of 'contact dermatitis of the hands' was 40.0 following exposure to dinitrochlorobenzene (DNCB, a known potent sensitiser), and that the relative risk for the same disease was only 3.0 following exposure to formaldehyde. A casual reader might be tempted to conclude that DNCB is the more important risk factor. Such a conclusion might be incorrect

Table 2. A hypothetical example illustrating how low-grade irritants such as washing-up liquid can account for a greater proportion of all irritant contact dermatitis cases than stronger irritants such as cutting fluids when prevalence of exposure is considered

	Irritant contact dermatitis*	
	cutting oils	washing-up liquid
Rate in exposed	10,000/10^5/year	3,000/10^5/year
Rate in unexposed	2,000/10^5/year	1,500/10^5/year
Relative risk (RR)	5.0	2.0
Attributable risk (AR)	8,000/10^5/year	1,500/10^5/year
Prevalence of exposure (P), %	8.0	50.0
Population attributable risk (PAR = AR × P)	160/10^5/year	750/10^5year
Population attributable risk fraction (PARF = PAR/overall population rate), %	8.0	37.5

* Refers to a general population sample of 100,000 where the overall rate of ICD is 2,000/10^5/year.

without consideration of the actual prevalence of exposure to DNCB and formaldehyde in the population under study. Thus, if one were referring to a random sample of adult men and women, it would be possible for formaldehyde to account for more cases of ACD because formaldehyde is a common exposure found in many household products, whereas exposure to DNCB might be a rare event confined to occupational exposure in one or two individuals. Clearly, if the population in question referred to employees of a chemical plant that distilled DNCB, where many people came into accidental direct contact with DNCB, then preventing contact with DNCB may become the overriding public health issue, since it is likely that most cases of ACD in this situation would be due to DNCB rather than formaldehyde.

Table 3. The prevention paradox

	Removal of exposure in the affected	
	population	individual
Rare exposure with high relative risk	small benefit	large benefit
Common exposure with low relative risk	large benefit	small benefit

Conclusions

From the examples given, it can be seen that the answer to the question 'Which risk measure is appropriate for my study?' will depend on the nature of the study. Studies which seek to determine an answer to the question 'How strong is the risk factor?' will need to estimate relative risk, whereas the answer to the question 'How important is the risk factor in this particular population?' will require some form of measure of population impact such as etiologic fraction. In relation to ICD and ACD, low-grade irritants or sensitisers which are found commonly in the environment may do more harm than potent but rare irritants or sensitisers simply because they affect more people [8, 9].

The public health approach requires the health of the population to be considered as a whole, as if it were a living organism in its own right. This can be a difficult concept to grasp because most physicians are trained to help their patients on an individual basis. Doctors may therefore have a large impact on the health of individuals, but they may confer little benefit to the health of populations [10]. Conversely, those involved in successful health prevention programmes seldom have the same feedback as physicians engaged in treating individuals, because they never know *which* individuals benefit from the intervention. In the absence of such personal gratification, public health physicians have to be content with the knowledge that the rate of disease in a given population has fallen as a result of their intervention, and their 'patient' (the population) is in a healthier state overall. The conflict between prevention of disease in individuals and populations with respect to relative risk and prevalence of exposure is summarised in table 3.

In addition to considering the appropriateness of risk measure for studies of contact dermatitis, the author has drawn attention to the importance of defining the population at risk when making public health decisions. The impact of contact dermatitis in the general population may be very different from that in occupational groups working in unusual environments.

References

1 Bradford-Hill A: The environment and disease: Association or causation? J Roy Soc Med 1965;58: 295–300.

2 Hennekens CH, Burning JF: Measures of disease frequency and association; in Mayrent SL (ed): Epidemiology in Medicine. Boston, Little, Brown, 1987, pp 54–98.

3 Morris JA, Gardner MJ: Calculating confidence intervals for relative risks, odds rations, and standardised rations and rates; in Gardner MJ, Altman DG (eds): Statistics with Confidence. London, BMJ Publishing, 1989, pp 50–63.

4 Doll R, Peto R: Mortality in relation to smoking: Twenty years' observations on male British doctors. Br Med J 1976;2:1525–1536.

5 Williams HC: Smoking and psoriasis. Br Med J 1994;308:428–429.

6 Coenraads P-J, Smit J: Epidemiology of contact dermatitis; in Burr ML (ed): Epidemiology of Clinical Allergy. Basel, Karger, 1993, vol 31; pp 29–48.

7 De Boer EM, van Ketel WG, Bruynzeel DP: Dermatoses in metal workers. Contact Dermatitis 1989;20:212–218.

8 Meding BE, Swanbeck G: Prevalence of hand eczema in an industrial city. Br J Dermatol 1987; 116:627–634.

9 Nielsen NH, Menné T: Allergic contact sensitisation in an unslelected Danish population. Acta Derm Venereol (Stockh) 1992;72:456–460.

10 Barker DJP, Rose G (eds): Epidemiology in Clinical Practice, (ed 2) London, Churchill-Livingstone, 1981, pp 4–11.

H.C. Williams, Dermatoepidemiology Unit, Queen's Medical Centre, University Hospital, Nottingham NG7 2UH (UK)

Elsner P, Lachapelle JM, Wahlberg JE, Maibach HI (eds): Prevention of Contact Dermatitis. Curr Probl Dermatol. Basel, Karger, 1996, vol 25, pp 18–27

QSAR Predictive of Contact Allergy: Scope and Limitations

Jurij J. Hostýnek[a], *Philip S. Magee*[b], *Howard. I. Maibach*[c]

[a] ETRI, Lafayette,
[b] BIOSAR, Vallejo, and
[c] UCSF, San Francisco, Calif., USA

Prior to large-scale development, production and commercialization of new chemicals, as well as adaptation of established organic compounds to new uses, their potential to cause hypersensitivity disease upon dermal or systemic exposure requires investigation as part of the overall assessment of their potential for adverse health effects, as allergenicity is now a well-recognized component in the overall toxicological profile of chemicals. In order to properly assess such risks to humans, identification of potential sensitizers currently involves the use of laboratory animals, is performed mostly in the guinea pig and in the mouse. However, conventional animal test methods used for risk assessment purposes are time consuming and costly, requiring a relatively large number of animals, and rely on a subjective evaluation of clinical results. With the use of fast-working computers and sophisticated statistical software, it now becomes possible to raise the level of such routine animal evaluation programs from unavoidable experimental and biological variables and subjective evaluation, onto a theoretical plane, where physicochemical properties and chemical reactivity can be addressed individually as factors which determine events such as allergic sensitization, taking place on the cellular level. Historic data and structural descriptors or alerts can be organized in the form of databases, making them amenable to statistical analysis. Quantitative structure activity relationship (QSAR), one such method which objectively describes the interaction between chemicals and biological systems, is now increasingly being used in the prediction of biological activity and a variety of toxicological endpoints, contact allergy (or allergic contact sensitization, ACD) among them [1, 2]. Hypersensitivity to chemicals appears to become a serious health problem for the general population, and particularly in the work environment it may well be the most incapacitating condition as a consequence of skin exposure to chemical agents [3]. Especially since no fully validated in vitro model to assess allergenic potential is available, the development of empirically derived, mechanistically based QSAR models thus holds the potential to becoming a valid alternative to extensive animal testing.

Development of Allergy Databases and Early QSAR Systems

Systematic development of comprehensive databases designed to assist in the detection or prediction of skin sensitisation potential of chemicals was started some 20 years ago, facilitated by computerized data entering, processing and retrieval. Notable among the early efforts were those by Ziegler (INPRET, Information on Predictive Tests) [4] and CCS Associates (CADES, Contact Allergens Database Evaluation System) [5], significant compendia of published data which reflect all aspects rendered public on the subject of delayed-type skin sensitization caused by small-molecular-weight chemicals. Particularly the searchable CADES database, a continuing argus surveying the open literature published since 1965, allows the computerized search for contact allergens by name, chemical structure, type of tests with pertinent experimental data and results, or number of cases reported in the medical literature.

At the same time, several efforts focused on mechanistic rationale of immunological activity, correlating structural elements with clinical expression of allergy. As early as 1935, Landsteiner and Jacobs [6] had connected the occurrence of hypersensitivity with protein reactivity to exogenous agents. In the several efforts that followed, structure-activity correlations focused on homologous series or narrowly defined classes of chemicals: sultones [7], diacrylates and dimethacrylates [8], aromatic amines [9], 3-alkanesulfonates [10], bromoalkanes [11], urushiol analogues [12], *p*-quinones [13], combining a limited number of criteria and mechanisms of action, such as molecular size [11–13], protein reactivity or relative alkylation index [7, 10].

In this latter period, an encompassing view correlating the formation of immunogenic non-self with protein reactivity was then compiled in a treatise by Dupuis and Benezra [14], which attained pivotal importance in all QSAR efforts that followed. Viewed from the chemists' perspective, the occurrence of non-self due to exogenous agents thereby becomes a rational process of facile systematic analysis by expert systems, and forms the foundation of all subsequent efforts aimed at rationalizing sensitization using QSAR. An outstanding example of a recent computerized system featuring as many as 50 structural alerts possibly related to protein reactivity is DEREK (Deductive Estimation of Risk from Existing Knowledge) [15]. Applicable to different toxicological endpoints and adapted also to prediction of skin sensitization through guinea pig maximisation data (GPMT), it is such an empirical expert system accessible remotely and in an interactive mode through the University of Leeds, UK. Still, while comprehensively addressing protein reactivity of haptens and prohaptens, factors which determine the diffusivity of chemicals through biological membranes such as the skin are not an integral part of such a model. An expert system rulebase alone does not render the entire picture that allows predicting the sensitizing potential of a material, nor does it address the problem of over-reactivity toward SC protein or water.

Factors Determining Diffusivity through the Stratum Corneum

A set of physicochemical parameters is used to characterize a given molecular structure, which determines its diffusivity and partitioning among the different bio-organic phases of membranes such as the SC. Identifying subtle differences in molecular structure, they are continuous descriptors serving to predict mechanistic behavior in the transport, binding and interaction of molecules.

Molecular size (polarizable volume) describes London forces (induced dipole moments) and is calculated by molecular fragment descriptors developed at BIOSAR [Magee, unpubl. study PM182: Estimation of MR Fragment Values, 1980]. The calculated values (MR, molar refraction) are colinear with molecular volume ($r = 0.97$).

The polarity of the permeant chemical dictates the permeation path through the stratum corneum (SC) and is expressed as the logarithm of its octanol-water partition $\log P_{oct}$. It is of critical importance in the case of very reactive chemicals, as reaction in the protein domain of the SC will generally prohibit further permeation and subsequent reaction with the Langerhans cells in the epidermis. Compounds of relatively high water solubility ($\log P_{oct}$ below 1.0) easily penetrate the protein domain of the SC and react with the protein before reaching the viable epidermis and becoming immunogenic. A large body of octanol-water partitioning values has been compiled by Hansch et al. [16] in the Pomona College Medicinal Chemistry Project (PCMCP) logP database. For compounds for which no experimental data exist, on the other hand, an accurate method (CLOGP) has been elaborated at the PCMCP for calculating logP by summation of fragment values. The value for logP in turn can be separated into a lipophilic increment, PL, and a hydrophilic contribution

PH, each again calculable by summation of incremental values assigned to subunits making up molecular structure [17]. For purposes of ACD potential, our group concluded that PL is a better descriptor than is logP.

H-bond donors (HBD) are obtained from a count of the N-H and O-H groups of the molecule, and H-bond acceptors (HBA) by a count of the electron pairs on oxygen and nitrogen. These numbers are adjusted downward for any intramolecular bonds, as these reduce the potential of the compound for protein binding. These numbers represent a potential for forming both types of H-bonds, and both can be significant.

The second type of descriptor, an indicator variable indentifying reactive sites (haptens) and potential for metabolism (pro-haptens) is based on structural alerts as determined by Dupuis and Benezra [14], with values of 1 or 0 to indicate the presence or absence of such features. This characterization of a molecule is most critical and highly dependent on chemical knowledge and experience, as opposed to a rigid computerized approach.

A Comprehensive ACD Classification Model

The heretofore missing aspect in characterizing barrier diffusivity was integrated into the analytical process which analyzed sensitization data for potential qualitative structure-activity relationships. Thus, a comprehensive algorithm was developed by our group which reflects protein reactivity and metabolism as well as skin penetration, the latter a prerequisite for any type of subsequent tissue reaction. This process of membrane diffusion and binding is determined by mechanistic descriptors of size, polarity and hydrogen bonding, expressed as continuous variables which can be calculated.

Development of the biologically based QSAR model proceeded through tabulation of descriptors from structural analysis of 35 compounds known to be severe-to-moderate contact allergens, and 36 non-allergens chosen among molecules of diverse structure and functionality, ranging in complexity from formaldehyde to steroids. Using the discriminant technique of two-value multiple regression analysis, through progressive elimination of descriptors with low statistical strength, a predictive model resulted that is based on five indicator variables and four continuous variables chosen from an initial set of 22. Within the model, the 71 allergens and nonallergens were adequately separated ($r=0.82$). Of the 35 allergens, 34 were correctly predicted (97% sensitivity), while identification of 33 of the 36 nonallergens was correct (92% specificity) [18].

For a first validation of this model, a further set of 38 allergens and 42 nonallergens not used in the learning set was then processed through the model. It showed a high degree of predictive power, yielding 84% concordance, 79% sensitivity (30/38) and 88% specificity (37/42) [19].

In vivo validation of the classification model was accomplished by matching its prediction against sensitization data obtained in the mouse. For that purpose, six chemicals selected at random and not previously investigated for allergenicity, were analyzed using the nine descriptors previously identified as significant in the model. The resulting classification was then matched with the results of the murine local lymph node assay (MLLNA) [11]. In the murine assay, all predicted allergens were confirmed as allergens at all concentrations, while 2 of the 3 predicted nonallergens were unreactive at all concentrations in the in vivo assay. One compound predicted as nonallergen had a negative response in the MLLNA at two concentrations, and a borderline response at one concentration [20].

A First Ranked ACD Model

Through the use of a modified statistical approach on a larger set of compounds, we strove to arrive at a first model which would not only identify the allergenic nature of a novel structure, but in case of positives also indicate the severity of a reaction to be expected. The predictive value of the first SAR model was to be raised from a yes/no classification to that of a predictive tool for the assessment of allergenic potency by analysis of a large ($n=88$) and diverse group of small nonelectrolytes ($-3<\log P<6$ and $40<MW<400$). Through resolution of clinical data on record, the relative potency of known allergens included in model construction was categorized in four distinct levels of ranking: non [29], weak [18], moderate [15] and strong [26]. Multiple regression analysis on these ranks (1–4) was performed starting out with the descriptors previously used to explore simple classification between allergens and non-allergens. Of those, the same 9 descriptors already seen in the classification model proved to be significant. The correlation achieved was statistically stronger than that of the previous, two-class problem ($r=0.84$). The substantial differences in molecular structure used in the two models provides further corroboration for the validity of those 9 key descriptors, as one study supports the other.

Discrimination between strong allergens and nonallergens achieved by this algorithm is perfect. As described by Gad [21], the prediction of a quantitative model based on the experimental spread of animal data can be $\pm$ 1 level (e.g. a '2' is correctly predicted in the range 1–3). Based on this criterion, concordance given by the first graded model is 100%. On the basis of exact match, the total concordance is 64%.

For validation of the graded model, a further set of 61 allergens and non-allergens not used in the learning set was processed through the model, showing concordance of 90% overall, and 97% for separation of inactives vs. strong allergens.

Multivariate QSAR analysis has thus proven effective in extracting mechanistic information in the process of developing predictive models which are based on subjective clinical assessments. The regression coefficients derived in this second stage again have direct physicochemical relevance to the percutaneous diffusion process, and confirm the results of earlier investigations. The predictive model thus derived represents an adequate, first algorithm for quantitative ACD risk assessment.

Limitations of the First Ranked Model

Certain limitations in utility inherent in this first graded model become evident upon examination of the clinical nature of data used in model construction. The data extracted from the literature were generated by different predictive protocols, using different models: human maximization test, mouse ear swelling test, murine local lymph node test, guinea pig maximization test, Freund's complete adjuvant test, etc. The model thus derived could not be considered predictive for any one particular species. Also, by restricting the choice of data to one species only when constructing an alternate graded model, an even better focus and thus concordance seemed a reasonable expectation. Survey of the literature reveals that an attempt towards building an exclusively human model would fail due to the paucity of useful, statistically meaningful data. The obvious alternative choice is the guinea pig, offering a wealth of test results, also generally accepted as a model of choice predictive of sensitization potential in man.

A Second Ranked ACD Model

Development of a model aiming to predict allergenic potential in man in a more focused manner was undertaken by applying severe criteria in data selection from the published literature. The past 20 years of experimental results pertaining to ACD were screened to exclude all but guinea pig data, and those which only used the GPMT and FCAT as predictive protocols. Statistically adequate sample sizes at the test and control stages were prerequisites, as was unequivocal identification and controlled purity of the chemicals used; only the highest sensitization scores were entered in the data base.

As in the first graded model, 77 inactives and allergens, graded by their relative potency, were categorized into four distinct levels of ranking and statistical analysis by four-level regression was again performed, eliminating all but the statistically relevant descriptors: 10 structural alerts (indicator variables), but only one continuous descriptor emerged as relevant from the analysis. This unexpected result, the apparent statistical irrelevance of continuous descriptors, as they serve to characterize molecular diffusivity through the SC barrier, seems to put into doubt the guinea pig as an appropriate model. It raises questions which are not easy to resolve, as one single answer alone may not address the entire scope of the problem. Does the guinea pig skin with its abundant hair follicles adequately model the barrier properties of human skin? Do the GPMT or FCAT tests in their prevailing mode of execution, intracutaneous injection of the test material for the induction phase, negate the protective function of the skin or the SC, intended to be a defense against ingress of exogenous agents? Is the topical challenge phase in particular the element which defeats the epidermal barrier function: open or occluded application of the test material on freshly shaven skin at an irritating concentration, in solvents such as alcohol or acetone; and with the case of non-irritants, on skin that has been pretreated with sodium lauryl sulfate to induce irritation?

Scope and Limitations of QSAR for ACD

From our critical examination of the literature, and in the process of structure analysis and coding for structural alerts towards a data base, a number of factors become apparent which seem to set serious limits to the predictive accuracy of a graded QSAR model which targets ACD, and even cast doubts on the benefits of a graded model. Some of these uncertainties, inherent in data analysis and model building, will be difficult to overcome as not all structural refinements can be coded for. Also accidental contaminants, reactivity, and, above all, metabolism (recognition of prohaptens) are some of the principal imponderables. Examples for uncertainty in coding are:

(1) Stereochemistry: Geraniol/nerol are stereo-isomers that code identically; yet in reality geraniol is a moderate sensitizer (confirmed in 4 different testing methods [22]) while nerol is inert.

(2) H-bonding: Donor-acceptor counts for methylsalicylate are not readily apparent; they are partially reduced due to internal H-bonding.

(3) Chirality: 1-Usnic acid is not allergenic, *d*-usnic acid is a moderate allergen [23].

(4) Contaminants: Pure *d*-limonene, long considered an allergen, is inactive; its readily formed epoxide (air oxidation) and its derivatives instead are allergens [24, 25].

Pure abietic acid, the main component of colophony, long considered the main allergen in the natural resin, is inactive [26, 27]. Readily air-oxidized, it converts to the potent allergen 15-hydroperoxyabietic acid [28].

(5) Metabolism: Cinnamic alcohol is a nonsensitizer in the guinea pig [29]; its metabolite, cinnamaldehyde, is a strong sensitizer [30].

(6) Diffusivity: Structural alerts that indicate allergenic potential are immunologically irrelevant in structures which will not penetrate beyond the SC due to their polarity or size, e.g. acrylate derivatives [31].

(7) Reactivity: Coumarin (aromatic B-ring) is inactive; dihydro coumarin is a reactive aromatic ester and reacts directly with SC protein [32]. Acrolein and glutaraldehyde are archetype allergens, yet appear inactive in the GPMT [33] and in man [34], as they react with SC protein before they can reach the epidermis.

(8) Overload effect: Alkylating agents can sensitize in a dose-dependent fashion, and desensitize beyond a threshold dose [7, 10].

(9) Dosing mode: Commonplace w/v dosing in animal testing overstates allergenicity of small-molecular weight chemicals [21].

Conclusions

Classification of chemicals as potential allergens vs. nonallergens by QSAR has proven successful. In the algorithm developed, many of the subtleties of metabolism and protein reactivity, which go beyond the artificial intelligence of so-called expert systems, are overlaid on transport and binding factors, and so are better able to distinguish between inherent sensitizing potential and the actual clinical expression of such reactivity. It could be demonstrated that for the diffusion process, lipophilic character, molecular size and both types of hydrogen bonding are important and that coding for protein reactivity or prohapten activation must proceed with full recognition of the molecular environment surrounding the substructure. Classification by QSAR appears attractive thanks to the advantage of presently available high computing capabilities, and is preferable to animal experimentation due to the fact that no material substance is required for this purely theoretical exercise, bringing an invaluable advantage to new drug discovery, among other fields of chemicals development. A conceptual or putative structure can hereby be analyzed in the model, before it is ever synthesized in the laboratory. Early business decisions and setting of priorities thus become possible before major project investments are necessary.

Development of ranked QSAR models for the accurate prediction of allergenic potency, on the other hand, appears handicapped by a number of factors: the principal ones being: (a) the quality of biological data on which a model forcibly is built; (b) the limited predictability of metabolism in the skin, and (c) the reactivity of certain structures which, under some circumstances, invite molecular orbital calculation before correct coding becomes possible.

Results achieved so far allow a clear separation between nonallergens and allergens, but only an approximation as to the severity of allergenic potential. By such semiquantitative assessment of sensitization risk, however, an early estimation of the risk/benefit ratio nevertheless becomes possible and is advantageous for agents which harbor the potential for therapeutic activity. Prioritisation and streamlining of the (drug) product development timeline, with corresponding reductions in costs and in the need for traditionally extensive laboratory animal testing undoubtedly comports a benefit in such an approach.

The construction of a human QSAR model must be excluded at this time due to the scarcity of statistically significant data, determined by the anecdotal nature of medical reports, and the ethical limits set for experimentation.

References

1 Hansch C, Dunn WJ III: Linear relationships between lipophilic character and biological activity of drugs J Pharm Sci 1972;61:1.

2 Hansch C, Leo A: Exploring QSAR: Fundamentals and Applications in Chemistry and Biology. ACS Professional Reference Book. Washington, American Chemical Society, 1995, vol 1.

3 Kanerva L, Jolanki R, Estlander T: Statistics on the causes of occupational contact urticaria and protein contact dermatitis. Allergologie 1995;18:473.

4 Ziegler V, Richter C, Ziegler B, Haustein U-F: INPRET-Database on Predictive Tests (Allergy). Semin Dermatol 1989;8:80–82.

5 Sigman CC, Bagheri D, Maibach HI: Approaches to structure-activity relationships in skin sensitization using CADES; in Rougier A, Goldberg AM, Maibach HI (eds): In vitro Skin Toxicology: Irritation, Phototoxicity, Sensitization. New York, Mary Ann Liebert, 1994, pp 271–280.

6 Landsteiner K, Jacobs J: Studies on the sensitization of animals with simple chemical compounds. J Exp Med 1935;61:643.

7 Roberts DW, Williams DL: The derivation of quantitative correlations between skin sensitization and physicochemical parameters for alkylating agents, and their application to experimental data for sultones. J Theor Biol 1982;99:807–825.

8 Roberts DW: Structure-activity relationships for skin sensitization potential of diacrylates and dimethacrylates. Contact Dermatitis 1987;17:281–289.

9 Benezra C, Sigman CC, Bagheri D, Holmes CT, Maibach HI: A systematic search for structure-activity relationships of skin sensitizers. II.*p*-Phenylenediamines. Semin Dermatol 1989;8:88–93.

10 Roberts DW, Fraginals R, Lepoittevin J-P, Benezra C: Refinement of the relative alkylation index (RAI) model for skin sensitization and application to mouse and guinea-pig test data for alkyl alkanesulphonates. Arch Dermatol Res 1991;283:387–394.

11 Basketter DA, Roberts DW, Cronin M, Scholes EW: The value of the local lymph node assay in quantitative structure-activity investigations. Contact Dermatitis 1992;27:137–142.

12 Roberts DA, Benezra C: Quantitative structure-activity relationships for skin sensitization potential of urushiol analogues. Contact Dermatitis 1993;29:78–83.
13 Hausen BM, Heitsch H, Borrmann B, Koch D, Rathmann R, Richter B, et al: Structure-activity relationships in allergic contact dermatitis. Contact Dermatitis 1995;33:12–16.
14 Dupuis G, Benezra C: Allergic Contact Dermatitis to Simple Chemicals. New York, Marcel Dekker, 1982.
15 Sanderson DM, Earnshaw CG: Computer prediction of possible toxic action from chemical structure: The DEREK system. Human Exp Toxicol 1991;10:261–273.
16 Hansch C, Leo A, Hoekman D: Exploring QSAR-Hydrophobic, Electronic, and Steric Constants. ACS Professional Reference Book. Washington, ACS, 1995, vol 2.
17 Magee PS: Complex factors in hydrocarbon/water, soil/water and fish/water partitioning. Sci Tot Envir 1991;109/110:155–178.
18 Magee PS, Hostýnek JJ, Maibach HI: A classification model for allergic contact dermatitis. Quant Structure-Activity Relat 1994;13:22–33.
19 Magee PS, Hostýnek JJ, Maibach HI: Modeling allergic contact dermatitis; in Rougier A, Goldberg AM, Maibach HI (eds): In vitro Skin Toxicology: Irritation, Phototoxicity, Sensitization. New York, Mary Ann Liebert, 1994, pp 281–291.
20 Hostýnek JJ, Lauerma AI, Magee PS, Bloom E, Maibach HI: A local lymph-node assay validation study of a structure-activity relationship model for contact allergens. Arch Dermatol Res 1995;287: 567–571.
21 Gad SC: A scheme for the prediction and ranking of relative potencies of dermal sensitizers based on data from several systems. J Appl Toxicol 1988;8:361–368.
22 Klecak G, Geleik H, Frey JR: Screening of fragrance materials for allergenicity in the guinea pig. Comparison of four testing methods. J Soc Cosmet Chem 1977;28:53–64.
23 Mitchell JC, Shibata S: Immunologic activity of some substances derived from lichenized fungi. J Invest Derm 1969;52:517–520.
24 Karlberg A-T, Magnusson K, Nilsson U: Air oxidation of *d*-limonene (the citrus solvent) creates potent allergens. Contact Dermatitis 1992;26:332–340.
25 Karlberg A-T, Shao LP, Nilsson U, Gafvert E, Nilsson JLG: Hydroperoxydes in oxidized d-limonene identified as potent contact allergens. Arch Dermatol Res 1994;286:97–103.
26 Karlberg A-T, Bergstedt E, Boman A, Bohlinder K, Lidén C, Nilsson G, et al: Is abietic acid the allergenic component of colophony. Contact Dermatitis 1985;13:209–215.
27 Karlberg A-T: Pure abietic acid is not allergenic. Contact Dermatitis 1989;21:282–286.
28 Karlberg A-T, Bohlinder K, Boman A, Hacksell U, Hermansson J, Jacobsson S, et al: Identification of 15-hydroperoxyabietic acid as a contact allergen in Portuguese colophony. J Pharm Pharmacol 1988;40:42–47.
29 Sharp DW: The sensitization potential of some perfume ingredients tested using a modified Draize procedure. Toxicology 1978;9:261–271.
30 Weibel H, Hansen J, Andersen KE: Cross-sensitization patterns in guinea pigs between cinnamaldehyde, cinnamyl alcohol and cinnamic acid. Acta Derm Venereol (Stockh) 1989;69:302–307.
31 Ashby J, Hilton J, Dearman RF, Kimber I: Streptozotocin: Inherent but not expressed skin sensitizing potential. Contact Dermatitis 1995;33:165–167.
32 Hausen BM, Schmieder M: The sensitizing capacity of coumarins (I). Contact Dermatitis 1986; 15:157–163.
33 Susten AS, Breitenstein MJ: Failure of acrolein to produce sensitization in the guinea pig maximization test. Contact Dermatitis. 1990;22:299–300.
34 Maibach HI, Prystowsky SD: Glutaraldehyde (pentanedial) allergic contact dermatitis. Arch Dermatol 1977;113:170–171.

Jurij J. Hostýnek, 3644 Happy Valley Rd., Lafayette, CA 94549 (USA)

Elsner P, Lachapelle JM, Wahlberg JE, Maibach HI (eds): Prevention of Contact Dermatitis. Curr Probl Dermatol. Basel, Karger, 1996, vol 25, pp 28–36

In vitro Sensitization of Human T Cells with Hapten-Treated Langerhans Cells: A Screening Test for the Identification of Contact Allergens

Maya Krasteva[a], *Corinne Moulon*[a], *Josette Péguet-Navarro*[a], *P. Courtellemont*[b], *G. Redziniak*[b], *D. Schmitt*[a]

[a] Laboratoire Peau Humaine et Immunité, INSERM U346, Hôpital Edouard-Herriot, Lyon, and

[b] Centre de Recherche PCD, Saint-Jean de Braye, France

The need to develop predictive tests to identify allergens and thus reduce the hazards resulting from occupational and consumer exposure to new products has been recognized for many years [1, 2]. Animal welfare movement and an increasing understanding of immunological mechanisms involved in contact sensitivity have prompted an accelerated development of in vitro testing methodologies. At present, the use of full in vitro human assays for the assessment of contact sensitivity responses has been limited chiefly to the study of strong sensitizers and peripheral blood mononuclear cells have been used as antigen-presenting cells (APC) [3, 4]. In a previous study we provided the first direct evidence for the ability of human Langerhans cells (LC) to sensitize in vitro naive T cells to a hapten (trinitrophenyl) [5]. The present study is aimed at testing the ability of a range of contact sensitizers to induce in vitro primary sensitization of autologous T cells using cultured human LC as APC.

Materials and Methods

Langerhans Cell-Enriched Epidermal Cell Suspensions

Epidermal cell suspensions were obtained from normal human skin (plastic surgery) by trypsinization. They were enriched in LC by density gradient centrifugation. Cells from the interface containing 10–18% LC were incubated for 48 h at 37 °C in complete medium supplemented with human recombinant granulocyte-macrophage colony-stimulating factor (GM-CSF). After incubation viable cells (cultured Langerhans cells; cLC: 15–28%) were recovered by density centrifugation. These LC were used as APC in the T-cell proliferative assays.

T Cells

Autologous T cells were isolated from peripheral blood as previously described [6].

Test Chemicals

The allergens chosen for the study were 2,4,6-trinitrobenzene sulfonic acid (TNP; Sigma) and fluorescein isothiocyanate (FITC; Sigma), known as strong contact allergens; *p*-phenylenediamine base (PPDA; Sigma), a weaker but still highly sensitizing agent and its oxidation product Bandrowski's base (BB; ICN); several fragrance materials with low contact sensitizing capacity: citronellal (Sigma), hydroxycitronellal (Janssen), coumarin (Sigma). An irritant, sodium dodecyl sulfate (SDS; Sigma), was used as control of hapten specificity. The working concentrations, including the highest nontoxic concentrations, were as follows: PPDA and BB 1–3 μg/ml; citronellal 5–50 μg/ml; hydroxycitronellal 5–10 μg/ml; coumarin 10–100 μg/ml; SDS 5–50 μg/ml. To circumvent problems related to toxicity of TNP and FITC, APC were haptenated before they were cultured with T cells. TNP modification was performed according to the method of Shearer [7]. The other chemicals were added directly to the cultures.

Lymphoproliferative Assays

The cells were cultured in round-bottomed microtiter plates (10^5 autologous T cells and graded numbers of 2-day-incubated LC in a final volume of 200 μl culture medium per well) at 37 °C in a humidified atmostphere of 5% CO_2 in air. The culture medium was RPMI-1640 supplemented with 10% heat-inactivated human AB serum, gentamicin, *L*-glutamine and indomethacin. Triplicate cultures for each allergen concentration were maintained for 3–5 days. A kinetic study of T-cell proliferation was performed by pulsing the cells with 1 μCi of ^{3}H-thymidine for the final 18 h of culture. Results from triplicate wells were expressed as mean cpm ± SD. Antigen-specific stimulation was calculated as stimulation indexes (SI = uptake of isotope in stimulated culture/uptake of isotope in nonstimulated culture). Statistical analyses were performed using Student's t test.

Results

Determination of the Optimal Conditions for Obtaining a Primary T-Cell Response in vitro

We analyzed the kinetics of the primary T-cell response induced by a graded number of TNP-treated fresh or 2-day incubated LC. T lymphocytes (10^5) were cultured 3–7 days with 10^3 to 8×10^3 LC per well. As previously reported [5], TNP-modified fresh LC did not induce a detectable lymphoproliferative response. By contrast, TNP-modified cLC generated a primary T-cell response which was the highest when 4×10^3 LC were cultivated with 10^5

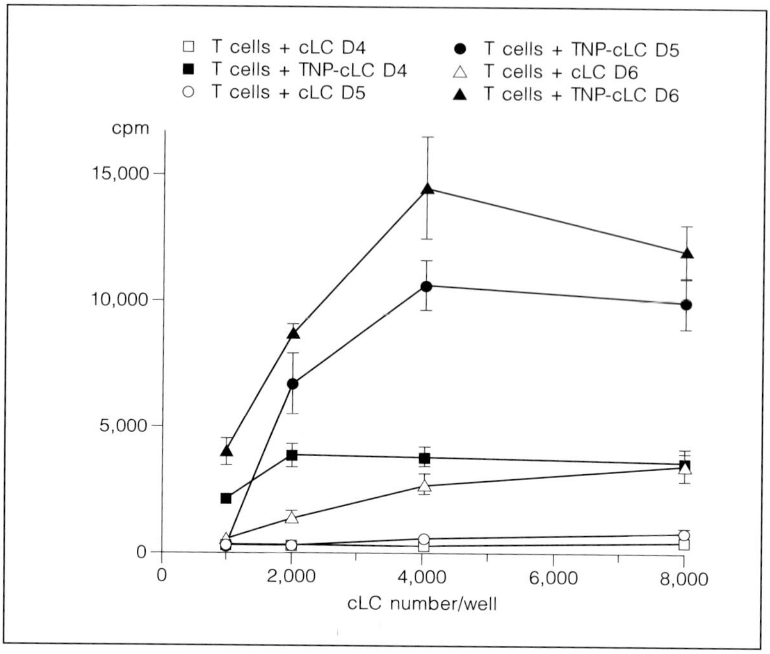

Fig. 1. In vitro primary T-cell response to a graded number of TNP-modified cLC. T lymphocytes (10^5) were cocultured with 2-day cLC, treated or not with TNP. T-cell proliferation was assessed at days 4 (D4), 5 (D5) or 6 (D6) by ^{3}H-thymidine incorporation for the final 18 h of culture. Results are expressed as mean cpm $\pm$ SD of triplicate cultures.

T cells (fig. 1). The autologous response to cLC was not significant and was proportional to the number of LC. The best stimulation indexes were recorded after 5 days of culture (SI = 20), but were significant at days 4 and 6 as well (SI = 13.3 and 6.2, respectively). Thereafter, we studied the T-cell response to the other chemicals by applying the conditions in which we had obtained the highest responses to TNP.

In vitro Primary T-Cell Response to Various Chemicals

We analyzed the in vitro proliferative T-cell response to cLC after treatment of these cells with various chemicals. We chose a stimulation index of 3 or greater as a criterion for the induction of primary sensitization. Data from a representative experiment are shown in figure 2a. Significant stimulation indexes were obtained with highly sensitizing chemicals (TNP and FITC). Weak sensitizers (coumarin, citronellal, hydroxycitronellal) did not induce a significant T-cell response. A stimulation index lower than 3 was obtained

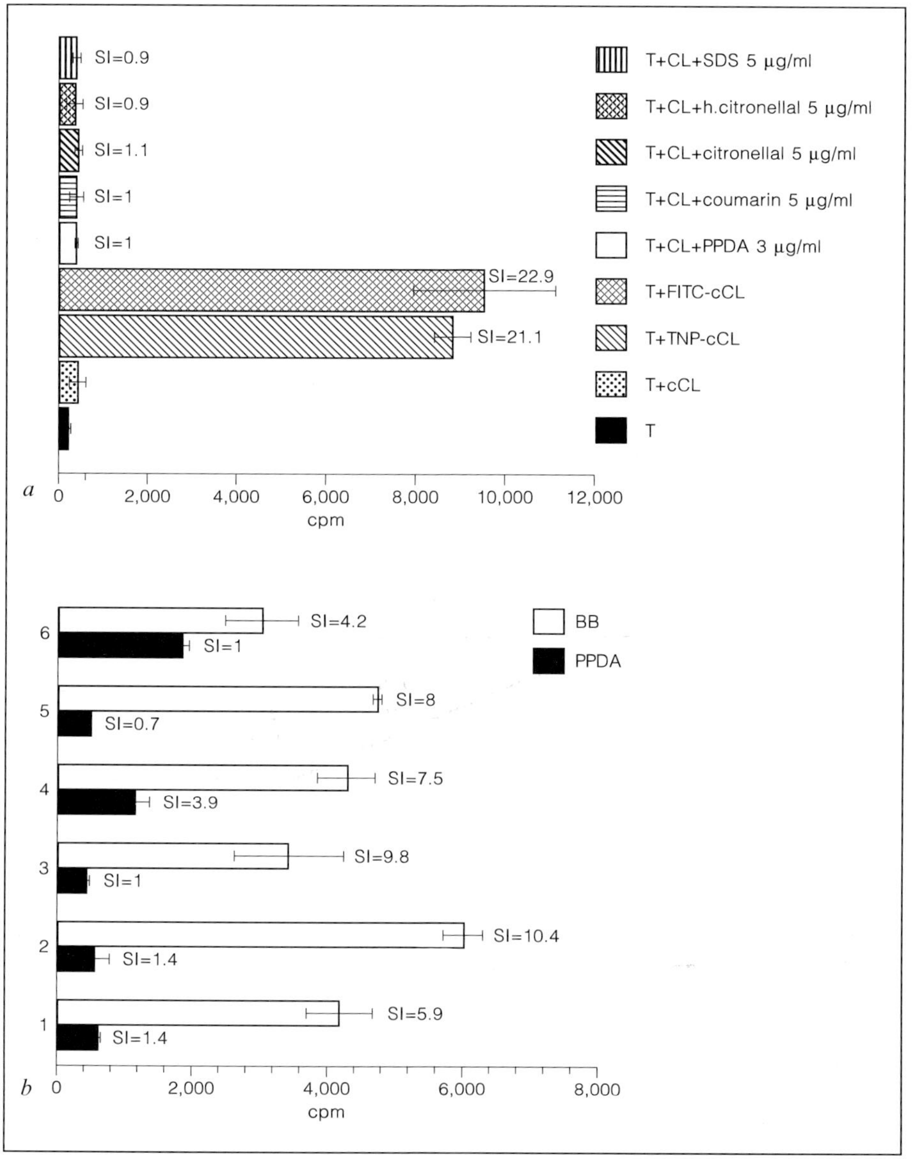

Fig. 2. Comparative in vitro T-cell-proliferative responses to various chemicals. T lymphocytes (10^5) were cocultured for 4–6 days with 2-day cLC. T-cell proliferation at day 5 was assessed by ^{3}H-thymidine incorporation during the final 18 h of culture. Results are expressed as mean cpm ± SD of triplicate cultures. Antigen-specific stimulation was calculated as stimulation indexes (SI = uptake of isotope in stimulated culture/uptake of isotope in nonstimulated control culture). *a* T-cell proliferative response at day 5 of culture in a representative experiment. *b* Highest proliferative responses to PPDA and BB in 6 experiments.

Table 1. Highest T-cell responses to chemically treated cLC

	TNP	FITC	Coumarin	Citronellal	Hydroxy-citronellal	PPDA	SDS
Number of experiments	13	10	12	10	8	6	10
Number of experiments in which a primary T-cell response was generated	13	7	1	0	2	1	0
Range of highest stimulation indexes	3.5–25.4	2.4–23.8	0.9–3.2	1.1–2.2	1.0–8.0	1.3–2.7	1.3–2.7
Mean stimulation indexes ± SD	12.8 ± 7.4	10.1 ± 8	1.8 ± 0.7	1.6 ± 0.4	2.6 ± 2.3	1.6 ± 1.2	1.8 ± 0.4

Antigen-specific stimulation was calculated as stimulation indexes (SI = uptake of isotope in stimulated culture/uptake of isotope in nonstimulated control culture).

with the irritant SDS. However, PPDA, a strong contact sensitizer, did not induce a significant lymphoproliferative response.

The calculation of stimulation indexes makes possible the comparison of the primary T-cell response induced by the different haptens in several experiments carried out with different donors. We have shown in table 1 the highest stimulation indexes registered within a single experiment. TNP induced primary sensitization in all 13 experiments and a dose-response relationship was observed. FITC failed to induce a primary in vitro response in only 3 of 10 experiments. T cells did not proliferate significantly to any working concentration of SDS and citronellal. The other haptens induced a significant T-cell proliferation in a limited number of experiments. The responses were, however, dose dependent and were the highest after 5 days of culture with coumarin (50 μg/ml) and PPDA (3 μg/ml) and after 6 days of culture with hydroxycitronellal (10 μg/ml).

In vitro Primary T-Cell Response to Bandrowski's Base

We have shown in a previous study that secondary proliferative responses of peripheral blood monocytes from patients sensitized to PPDA were higher when using BB, a metabolization product of PPDA, as a stimulating agent than when using PPDA itself [8]. We therefore compared the ability of BB and PPDA to induce a primary T-cell response in the present assay. As shown in figure 2b, BB generated significant T-cell proliferation in all experiments, while PPDA was effective in only 1 of 6 assays. BB generated the highest

T-cell responses after 6 days of culture and a dose-response relationship could be observed.

Statistical Analysis

The present in vitro model allows to differentiate strong contact allergens (TNP, FITC, BB) from weak allergens (coumarin, citronellal, hydroxycitronellal) and irritants ($p<0.05$). However, no significant differences were found between the stimulation indexes of weak allergens and an irritant (SDS).

Discussion

The present study was aimed at developing a model of in vitro priming of human naive T cells to contact allergens with different sensitizing potentials. The evaluation of in vitro hapten-induced primary proliferative responses in man provides an interesting alternative to animal testing, as it obviates the necessity of intra-species extrapolation. We have used in our model the cells that are physiologically involved in the generation of contact sensitivity response, i.e. T cells and LC. Furthermore, we have reproduced as far as possible the conditions necessary for functional in vitro maturation of LC. While the role of LC as APC is now firmly established, the importance of a short-term incubation of LC with GM-CSF has been reported only recently [9]. In a previous study we obtained for the first time an in vitro T-cell primary proliferative response to a hapten (TNP) using human LC as APC [5]. We found that LC incubated for 2 days in the presence of GM-CSF, but not fresh LC were able to sensitize T cells to TNP, thus confirming the results obtained by Hauser and Katz [10] in a murine model. In the present study, we induced primary sensitization to TNP in all 13 experiments. We were able to generate a primary response to FITC in 7 of 10 experiments. FITC has been shown to induce in vitro primary sensitization of murine responder lymph node cells using as APC syngeneic dendritic cells [11]. More recently, Hauser et al. [12] reported in vitro priming of Th cells by FITC-modified murine LC. To our knowledge in vitro sensitization to FITC using human LC as APC has never been generated before.

PPDA is ranked as a strong to extreme sensitizer in all in vivo predictive tests [13, 14]. It produced a significant proliferative response in our in vitro model in only 1 of 6 experiments. However, BB, an oxidation product of PPDA, induced primary sensitization in all the experiments. We have previously shown that BB induced a dose-dependent secondary proliferative response of peripheral blood mononuclear cells obtained from patients contact sensitive to PPDA which was higher than the response to PPDA itself [8]. We thus provided experimental evidence to the concept of PPDA being the prohapten in PPDA contact sensitivity [15] and suggested that BB could be the immunogenic hapten. The failure to induce reproducible primary sensitization to PPDA in the present in vitro system confirms that assumption. We are aware that contact allergy is a reaction involving several organ systems and that it is impossible to develop an in vitro model that could reflect all the complex reactions taking place from the moment in which the allergen is applied on the skin to the appearance of skin lesions. A limitation of our model is that it cannot reproduce the metabolisation in the dermis of certain chemical compounds, designated as prohaptens to immunogenic moieties. Therefore, it is representative of phenomena occurring in a definite compartment of the contact sensitivity reaction after the chemical has penetrated in the skin and has undergone modification by enzyme systems in as yet unknown compartment.

Coumarin, citronellal and hydroxycitronellal are widely used fragrance materials. The failure of citronellal to induce primary T-cell sensitization in our assay is in accordance with the negative results from human predictive testing [16] and reported epidemiologic data. Coumarin induced a significant lymphoproliferative response in 1 of 12 experiments. Although a human maximization test with coumarin did not sensitize anyone in a group of 25 volunteers [17], case reports of contact sensitization can be found in the literature and therefore we consider the results of our in vitro test concerning coumarin as relevant to its capacity to generate contact sensitizaion in vivo. Hydroxycitronellal has been identified as one of the causes of allergic contact dermatitis from household and personal care products and has been included in the fragrance mix of the European standard patch test series. There is a discrepancy between the results from a number of predictive studies carried out on humans revealing a very low potential for human sensitization [18] and the results obtained in animal models which rank it as a moderate sensitizer [14]. It induced a significant T-cell response only in a couple of experiments in our study. This reflects the conflicting results from human and animal predictive tests and patch test data. Two possibilities could be considered to explain that coumarin and hydroxycitronellal induce in vitro primary sensitization only in a limited number of experiments. First of all, in the light of the prohapten concept, they might be metabolized, like PPDA, to other products which would be able to induce a constant and dose-dependent T-cell response. Their failure to induce primary sensitization in the majority of the experiments might be also attributed to MHC restriction of the immune response.

SDS has been used as a model chemical for studying the skin response to irritant insult [19]. While it has never been shown to elicit contact sensitivity in human volunteers or in the guinea pig model [1, 2], it was reported to produce false-positive results in the local lymph node assay [20, 21]. SDS has been shown to cause LC migration from the epidermis to the draining lymph nodes, presumably by stimulating the production of TNF-α by keratinocytes and it has been suggested that these migrating LC bear 'environmental antigens' which induce a proliferative response [22]. In the present in vitro model SDS did not induce a significant T-cell proliferation in any of the experiments. This assay therefore provides better control of test conditions, with no interference of extrinsic factors such as 'environmental allergens'.

In conclusion, we presented here an in vitro model of human T-cell sensitization by hapten-treated cLC. This model allows discrimination between two groups of substances: strong contact sensitizers (TNP, FITC, BB) and weak sensitizers (coumarin, citronellal, hydroxycitronellal) and irritants (SDS). It cannot discriminate between weak sensitizers and irritants, nor can it predict the sensitizing potential of prohaptens. An important advantage of our in vitro model is that it does not overestimate the sensitizing potential of irritant substances. It could be used as a screening in vitro assay to eliminate strong contact allergens before further predictive animal tests have to be performed.

References

1 Kligman AM: The identification of contact allergens by human assay. III. The maximization test: A procedure for screening and rating contact sensitizers. J Invest Dermatol 1966;47:393–409.

2 Magnusson B, Kligman AM: The identification of contact allergens by animal assay: The guinea pig maximization test. J Invest Dermatol 1969;52:268–276.

3 Seldin MF, Rich RR: Human immune responses to hapten-conjugated cells. I. Primary and secondary proliferative responses in vitro. J Exp Med 1978;147:167–178.

4 Charmot D, Mawas C: The in vitro cellular response of human lymphocytes to trinitrophenylated autologous cells: HLA D restriction of proliferation but apparent absence of HLA restriction of cytolysis. Eur J Immunol 1979;9:723–728.

5 Moulon C, Péguet-Navarro J, Courtellemont P, Redziniak G, Schmitt D: In vitro primary sensitization and restimulation of hapten-specific T cells by fresh and cultured human epidermal Langerhans' cells. Immunology 1993;80:373–379.

6 Péguet-Navarro J, Dalbiez-Gauthier C, Dezutter-Dambuyant C, Schmitt D: Dissection of human Langerhans cells' allostimulatory function: The need for an activation step for full development of accessory function. Eur J Immunol 1993;23:376–381.

7 Shearer GM: Cell mediated cytotoxicity to trinitrophenyl-modified syngeneic lymphocytes. Eur J Immunol 1974;4:527–532.

8 Krasteva M, Nicolas JF, Chabeau G, Garrigue JL, Bour H, Thivolet J, Schmitt D: Dissociation of allergenic and immunogenic functions in contact sensitivity to para-phenylenediamine. Int Arch Allergy Immunol 1993;102:200–204.

9 Romani N, Lenz A, Glassel H, Stossel H, Stanzl U, Majdic O, Fritsch P, Schuler G: Cultured human Langerhans cells resemble lymphoid dendritic cells in phenotype and functions. J Invest Dermatol 1989;93:600–606.

10 Hauser C, Katz SI: Generation and characterization of T-helper cells by primary in vitro sensitization using Langerhans cells. Immunol Rev 1990;117:67–72.

11 Macatonia SE, Edwards AJ, Knight SC: Dendritic cells and the initiation of contact sensitivity to fluorescein isothiocyanate. Immunology 1986;59:509–514.

12 Hauser C, Yokoyama WM, Katz SI: Characterization of primary T helper cell activation and T helper cell lines stimulated by hapten-modified cultured Langerhans cells. J Invest Dermatol 1989; 93:649–655.
13 Marzulli FN, Maibach HI: The use of graded concentrations in studying skin sensitizers: Experimental contact sensitization in man. Food Cosmet Toxicol 1974;12:219–227.
14 Basketter DA, Scholes EW: Comparison of the local lymph node assay with the guinea pig maximization test for the detection of a range of contact allergens. Food Chem Toxicol 1992;30:65–69.
15 Dupuis G, Benezra C: Allergic Contact Dermatitis to Simple Chemicals. New York, Dekker, 1982.
16 Opdyke DLJ: Monographs on fragrance raw materials. Food Cosmet Toxicol 1975;13:681–923.
17 Opdyke DLJ: Monographs on fragrance raw materials. Food Cosmet Toxicol 1974;13:517–593.
18 Ford RA, Api AM, Suskind RR: Allergic contact sensitization potential of hydroxycitronellal in humans. Food Chem Toxicol 1988;26:921–926.
19 Widmer J, Elsner P, Burg G: Skin irritant reactivity following experimental cumulative irritant contact dermatitis. Contact Dermatitis 1994;30:35–42.
20 Basketter DA, Scholes EW, Kimber I: The performance of the local lymph node assay with chemicals identified as contact allergens in the human maximization test. Food Chem Toxicol 1994;32:543–547.
21 Montelius J, Wahlquist H, Boman A, Fernstrôm P, Grabergs L, Wahlberg JE: Experience with the murine local lymph node assay: Inability to discriminate between allergens and irritants. Acta Derm Venereol 1994;74:22–27.
22 Cumberbatch M, Kimber I: Tumour necrosis factor-α is required for accumulation of dendritic cells in draining lymph nodes and for optimal contact sensitization. Immunology 1995;84:31–35.

J. Péguet-Navarro, INSERM U346, Pavillon R, Hôpital Edouard-Herriot,
F–69437 Lyon Cedex 03 (France)

Elsner P, Lachapelle JM, Wahlberg JE, Maibach HI (eds): Prevention of Contact Dermatitis. Curr Probl Dermatol. Basel, Karger, 1996, vol 25, pp 37–46

Cutaneous Microdialysis for the Measurement in vivo of the Percutaneous Absorption of Organic Solvents

C. Anderson[a], *T. Andersson*[a], *A. Boman*[b], *M. Molander*[b]

[a] Department of Dermatology, University Hospital, Linköping;
[b] Department of Occupational Dermatology, National Institute of Occupational Health, Solna, and
[c] Vadstena Kemanalys, Vadstena, Sweden

Exposure to organic solvents is an important occupational problem since these agents have the potential to induce both systemic toxicity and contact dermatitis [1–3]. As regards systemic toxicity, although the respiratory route generally receives more attention, percutaneous penetration can at times be of greater consequence (fig. 1) [4].

Microdialysis is a bioanalytical sampling technique, which can be used to measure endogenous and exogenous substances in vivo in a target tissue [5, 6]. Cutaneous microdialysis (the application of the technique to dermatological questions) has only recently been used for in vivo human studies [7]. In principle, the technique can be applied in three ways; use of the microdialysis tubing per se [8, 9]; transcutaneous microdialysis [10] or the concentric (manufactured) microdialysis probe [11] which we have used in our group. In this method of cutaneous microdialysis, the dialysis membrane at the tip of a probe is placed via a guide into the skin, 2–3 cm from the point of insertion, at a depth of around 1 mm [12]. The standard dialysis membrane used in our group is permeable to substances with a molecular weight of up to 20 kD. Using an alternative membrane, the ultrafiltration membrane, with a molecular weight cut-off of 100 kD, even larger molecules can be measured [13, 14]. We have studied two main areas – percutaneous absorption [15], which will be illustrated in the present article, and cutaneous inflammation. In the latter area, we have used histamine as the model inflammatory mediator [16]. Fig. 2

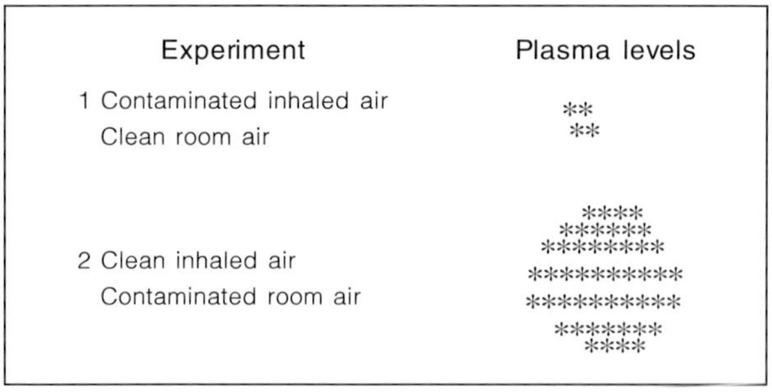

Fig. 1. In an experimental situation in which the relative importance (as reflected by plasma levels) of clean air exposed to the skin and clean inhaled air are compared, the potential for percutaneous absorption of 2-buthoxyethanol is illustrated [4].

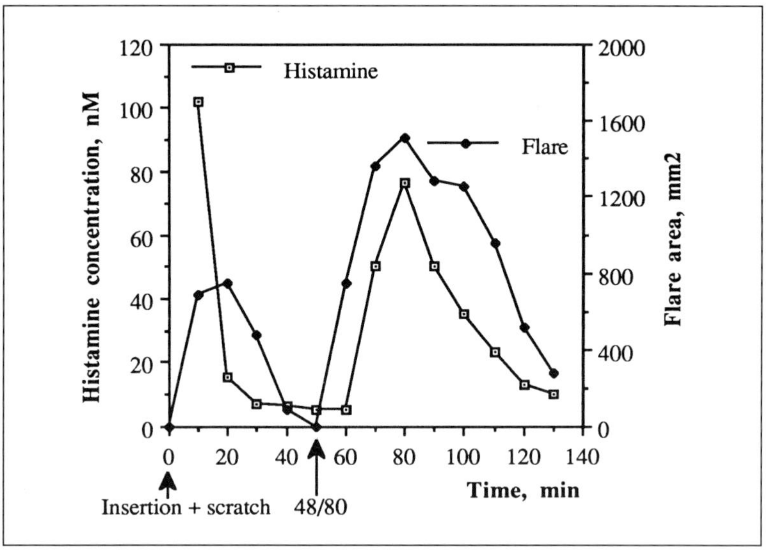

Fig. 2. Relationship between macroscopic flare response (mm^2) and histamine values (n*M*) in a healthy subject, provoked with compound 48/80, a known histamine-releasing agent.

shows the flare and histamine release after insertion of the probe and subsequent provocation with compound 48/80, a known histamine liberator. Cutaneous microdialysis, in contrast to the biopsy and suction blister technique, the previous alternatives for following a pharmacological course in the skin, does not preclude the use of multiparameter assessment of skin reactions, e.g. the use of laser Doppler perfusion imaging [17, 18].

Table 1. The general method of cutaneous microdialysis

I	Subject recruitment
II	Selection of skin site
	– Experimental skin site
	– Probe insertion site
III	Local anaesthesia
	– Skin entry site
IV	Insertion
	– Guide
	– Probe
V	Ultrasound assessment of probe depth
VI	Equilibration period
VII	Application of substance/provocation
VIII	Microdialysis sampling
IX	Sample analysis

The aim of the present study was to demonstrate the use of cutaneous microdialysis for the measurement of the percutaneous absorption of ethanol and isopropanol after topical application in excess to the skin of the ventral forearm in human volunteers.

Materials and Methods

Microdialysis Equipment

The essentials for the performance of microdialysis are a probe (containing the dialysis membrane), a pump and a collection system.

Probes. The standard microdialysis probe used (CMA/10, CMA/ Microdialysis Research AB, Sweden) has a shaft length of 70 mm and a membrane length of 10 mm. The steel shaft of the probe has an outer diameter of 0.64 mm. The diameter at the tip of the probe, where the polycarbonate or polyamide dialysis membrane is located, is 0.5 mm. The molecular weight cut-off point for the standard membrane is 20 kD. In some patients, a developmental flexible probe equipped with a polyamide membrane has been used.

Pump and Sample Collector. The perfusate was pumped by a CMA/100 microinjection pump. In some experiments when samples were to be collected over a longer period of time, a portable pump was used (CMA Microdialysis AB, Stockholm, Sweden). For sample collection, an automated collector (CMA/140 microfraction collector) synchronized with the pump was used. When the portable pump was used, manual collection of samples was performed.

General Method

The general method of human in vivo cutaneous microdialysis is shown in table 1.

Subject Recruitment. The in vivo experimentation was performed on human volunteers, all duly informed of the experimental conditions. The healthy volunteers were recruited mainly from departmental staff and the patients from the dermatology ward. The studies were approved by the regional ethics committee for human research, Linköping University Hospital.

Selection of Skin Site. The skin of the ventral forearm was selected as a suitable site for experimentation, usually the volar nonhairy midpart of the forearm. In all subjects, the tested skin looked normal to the naked eye. The intended position of the probe tip and the site of insertion, 3 cm apart, were marked with a small dot of ink. The site of guide insertion and subsequent probe position was chosen so as to avoid obvious veins. In experiments where two probes were used simultaneously, the tips of the probes were placed at least 3 cm apart.

Local Anesthesia. The skin entry site was anesthetized with local anesthetic (mepivacaine 5 mg/ml or lidocaine 10 mg/ml) which was injected intradermally to produce a bleb, approximately 3 mm in diameter. Guide insertion can also be performed without prior anesthesia.

Insertion. Use of a guide during insertion was necessary in order to protect the sensitive probe tip area. Two similar types of apheresis needles, Terumo 1.60×32 mm or Baxter 1.60×25 mm, were used. The guide was inserted parallel to the surface of the skin, the first part subcutaneously, the last centimeter corresponding to the subsequent location of the dialysis membrane, as superficially as possible. The probe was introduced through the entire length of the guide, which was then withdrawn, and taped in position. The probe tip thus lay at a distance of 32 or 25 mm, depending on the guide used, from the site of insertion.

Ultrasound Assessment of Probe Depth. The exact positioning of the probe during insertion can only be steered to a certain degree, the ultimate probe depth varying from 0.3 (the superficial dermis) to 2 mm (the subcutis), but usually being less than 1 mm. Ultrasound technique (Dermascan A, Sonatron AB, Sweden) has been used in most experiments in order to establish the possible influence of probe depth on microdialysis results.

Equilibration Period. The tissue trauma caused by the insertion procedure necessitates the use of a tissue equilibration period prior to subsequent experimentation. Based on histamine studies, a suitable equilibration period for histamine is at least 40 min [16]. Changes in skin blood perfusion after probe insertion, visualized by laser Doppler perfusion imaging, indicate a blood perfusion equilibration period of around 60 min [17]. For each individual target substance and experimental design, however, a new consideration of appropriate equilibration time should be performed. In the present study an equilibration time of around 30 min has been used.

Application of Solvents. A circular glass reservoir with an inner diameter of 15 mm and a depth of 8 mm was placed on the skin over the dialysis membrane and held in place by tape or glued (Casco synt-X Gel, cyanoacrylate glue) to the skin. The reservoir was filled with 99.5% ethanol or 100% isopropanol. The tape, or a glass cover slip glued to the reservoir as a cap, prevented evaporation (fig. 3). The ethanol was thus applied in excess to the skin for variable periods of up to 140 min, apart from two experiments in which the application period lasted 240 and 480 min.

Analysis of Ethanol and Other Solvents. In the analysis of solvents in earlier work [15], ethanol in the perfusate was analyzed (Vadstena Kemanalys, Vadstena, Sweden) by gas chromatography using a flame-ionisation detector system and a packed Porapac Q column. The lowest detectable ethanol level was approximately 3 μg/ml. In subsequent work, ethanol was analyzed by either of two methods: (1) according to a head space technique (Arbetsmiljöinstitutet, Solna, Sweden) [18] or (2) according to a direct injection method (Vadstena Kemanalys, Vadstena, Sweden), the latter method also being used in the analysis of isopropanol.

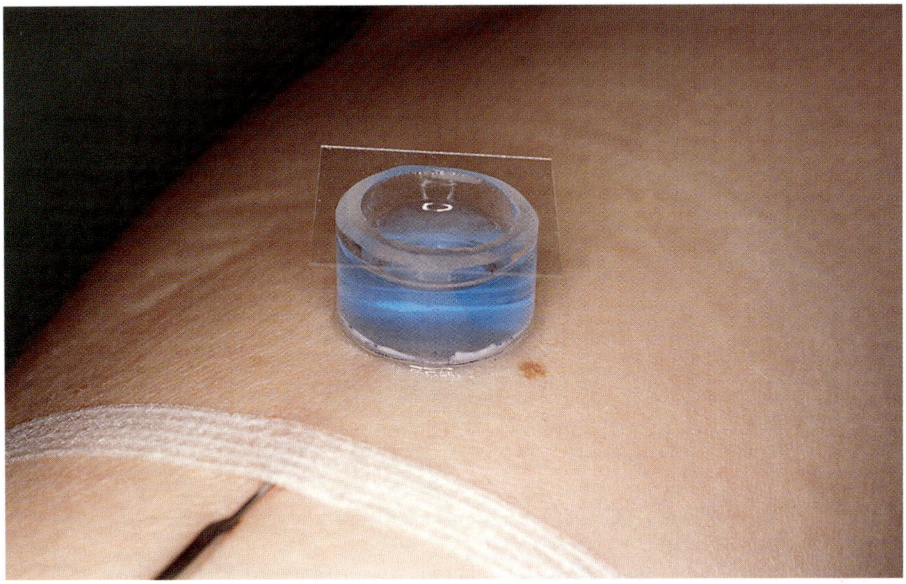

Fig. 3. Solvent application. The glass reservoir glued to the skin over the probe tip. The reservoir is filled with the solvent (in this illustration a blue dye has been added). A glass cover slip, glued to the reservoir prevents evaporation.

Results

We have found the cutaneous microdialysis procedure to be well tolerated by subjects. Probe insertion through anesthetized skin is painless but 'tunnelation' to the probe tip area can cause slight pain, which is usually well tolerated. Apart from occasional eccymoses, we have not encountered side effects.

In vitro, the dialysis membrane demonstrated good recovery characteristics for ethanol and isopropanol 0.01% in water both as single solutions and mixed. Using alternate ethanol and histamine recovery, no membrane damage could be demonstrated at relevant solvent concentrations.

In vivo, for both ethanol and isopropanol, levels could be detected in the dialysate within 20 min of application in all subjects. Figure 4 shows the results for isopropanol in a patient followed for 70 min after solvent application.

For practical reasons patients were followed for variable times after solvent application. Maximal levels seemed to occur at about 100 min after application, whereafter levels reached a plateau or fell. Figure 5 shows the results for

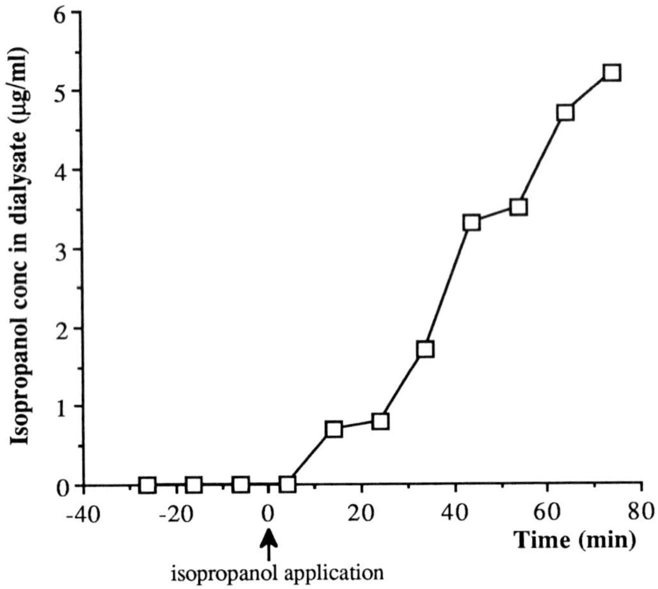

Fig. 4. Percutaneous absorption of isopropanol, continuously applied in excess to the skin over the dialysis probe. A 10-mm polyamide membrane was used. The flow rate was 3 µl/min.

ethanol in 1 patient. In experiments in which a portable pump was used, the levels reached a steady state in the period after 100 min.

Levels detected showed variability between subjects – probe depth seems to be the most important factor. Figure 6 illustrates the effect of probe depth in an experiment in which 2 probes were inserted in the same forearm in the same patient, one being more deeply placed than the other.

Discussion

Cutaneous microdialysis is a new in vivo technique in which the total human bibliography has expanded since first reports in 1991 and 1992 [15, 16, 19] but still comprises less than 20 reports. It is therefore hardly surprising that many practical and technical questions remain to be solved. The technique has come farthest in the study of cutaneous inflammation [7].

Our experience after using the technique since 1989 is that the procedure is well tolerated by patients. We have encountered no serious side effects. Using

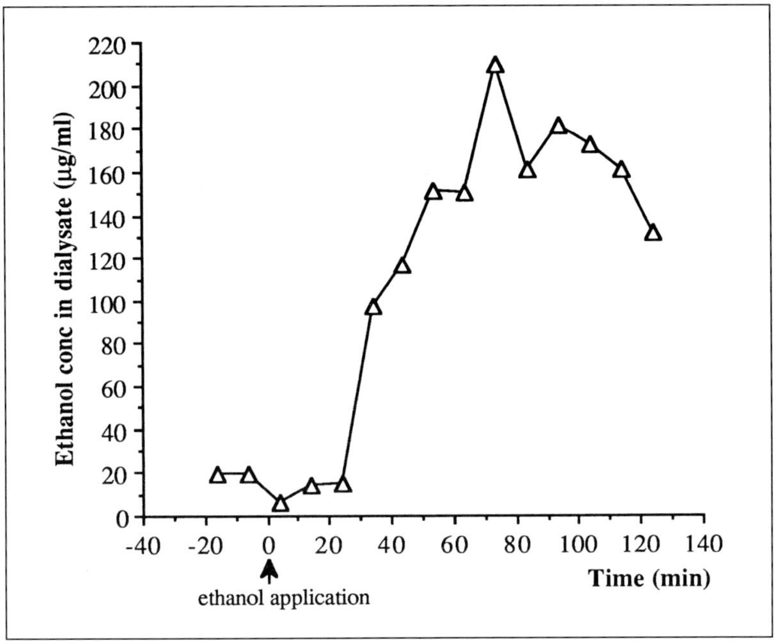

Fig. 5. Percutaneous absorption of ethanol in a male subject. Probe depth 0.8 mm. 99.5% ethanol was continuously applied in excess in a glass chamber on the skin over the dialysis probe in the skin of the ventral forearm. A 10-mm dialysis membrane was used, and the flow rate was 3 µl/min.

the standard (low-molecular-weight cut-off) microdialysis membrane smaller molecules can be studied. The ultrafiltration membrane (100 kD cut-off) is somewhat more difficult technically but can be used in the study of larger molecules [13]. The 100-kD cut-off probe has recently become commercially available (CMA Microdialysis AB, Stockholm, Sweden).

Percutaneous absorption has been defined as the penetration of substances from the outside into the skin and thereafter through the skin and into the blood and lymph vessels [20]. In cutaneous microdialysis, substances are measured in the dermal extracellular fluid, a compartment which, with earlier techniques, has not been accessible for investigation. Still, we have used the term percutaneous absorption in our microdialysis studies because we consider it to be an adequate description of the process which we have studied.

The 20-kD dialysis membrane used in this study has good in vitro recovery characteristics for ethanol and isopropanol. It should be recalled, however, that for each new substance studied, recovery and other aspects of interaction must be investigated.

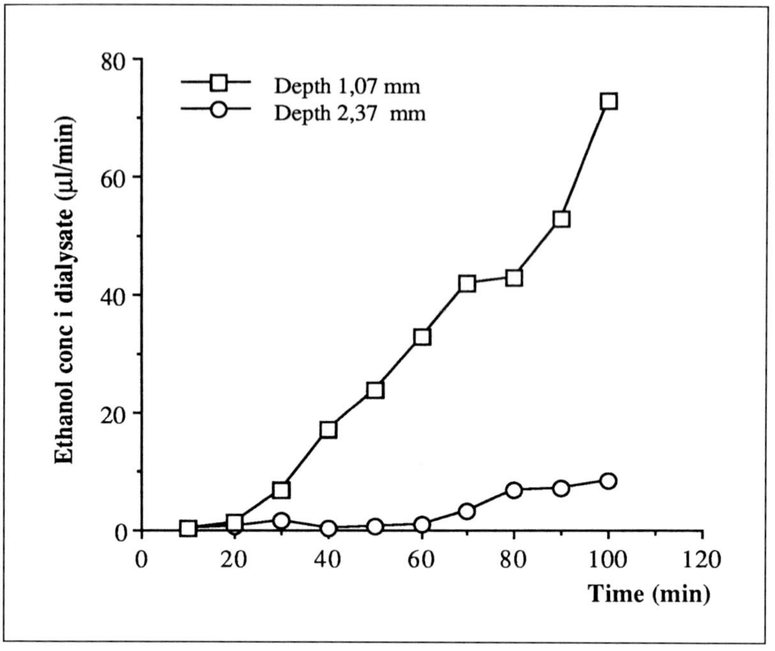

Fig. 6. Percutaneous ethanol absorption in two probes inserted in the skin of the ventral forearm of a 35-year-old healthy male. Probe membrane length was 5 mm and flow rate 3 µl/min.

An inter- and intraindividual variability in the levels of percutaneous absorption has been demonstrated. This has also been seen in nicotine studies performed with the same technique [21], and in our own studies of the percutaneous absorption of lidocaine and prilocaine from EMLA® cream [unpubl. data]. Probe depth seems to be the most important, but not the sole factor. Amongst the other aspects which need to be considered are constitutional and individual differences in barrier function, differences in tissue metabolic capacity and differences in tissue equilibration.

The present findings, which seem to support findings in the guinea pig in which a somewhat lower solvent plateau was reached after peak values [18], show the chronology of the percutaneous absorption – details of the pharmaco*kinetics* remain to be elucidated. Another area for development is modification of the perfusate for the study of lipophilic solvents (and other substances).

We consider cutaneous microdialysis to be a valuable technique for in vivo human studies of percutaneous absorption of a wide range of hazardous substances, including industrial solvents and pesticides. Even outside the area

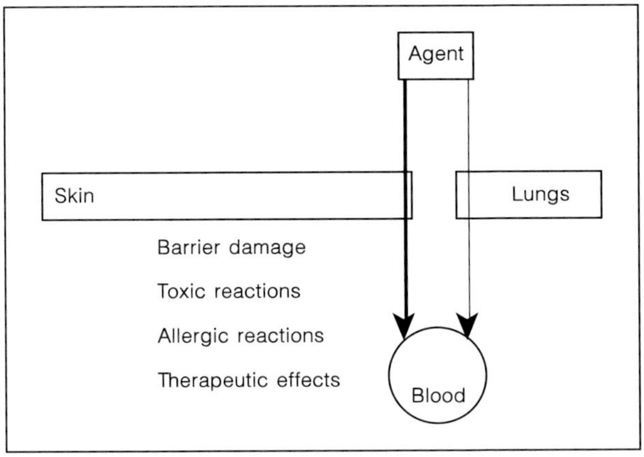

Fig. 7. Percutaneous absorption within the dermatological domain.

of toxicology and safety standards, however, an understanding of percutaneous absorption is important. In the pathogenesis of contact dermatitis, for instance, knowledge of skin penetration is relevant, as it is when topical therapy for dermatoses or transdermal delivery is used (fig. 7).

An important ethical and practical advantage in the study of potentially harmful agents, or in the study of locally applied therapeutic agents is that cutaneous microdialysis studies can be performed after the application of relatively small amounts of the agent to be studied. Previous techniques often precluded in vivo, human studies because of the need of test application over large areas or in high concentrations in order to manage distance analysis in blood or urine.

In summary, cutaneous microdialysis has been shown to be a promising technique for the study of the chronological course of inflammatory skin reactions. In the present study, the technique's possibilities for the in vivo human study of the pharmacokinetics of percutaneous absorption are demonstrated.

Acknowledgements

We are grateful for the expert assistance of Mrs. Catherine Svensson and Mrs. Florence Sjögren. These studies have been performed with financial assistance from the Swedish Work Environment Fund, the Swedish Association against Asthma and Allergy and the Edvard Welander Foundation.

References

1 Andersen KE: Systemic toxicity from percutaneous absorption of industrial chemicals; in Adams R (ed): Occupational Skin Disease. Philadelphia, Saunders, 1990, pp 73–88.
2 Boman A: Factors influencing the percutaneous absorption of organic solvents: An experimental study in the guinea pig. Arbete och Hälsa. Stockholm, National Institute of Occupational Health, 1989, vol 11, pp 1–51.
3 Boman A, Wahlberg JE: Percutaneous absorption of three organic solvents in the guinea pig. I. Effect of physical and chemical injuries to the skin. Contact Dermatitis 1989;21:36–45.
4 Johansson G, Boman A: Percutaneous absorption of 2-buthoxyethanol vapour in human subjects. Br J Ind Med 1991;48:788–792.
5 Ungerstedt U: Measurement of neurotransmitter release by intracranial dialysis; in Marsden CA (ed): Measurement of Neurotransmitter Release in vivo. Bath, Wiley, 1984, pp 81–105.
6 Ungerstedt U: Microdialysis: Principles and applications for studies in animals and man. J Intern Med 1991;230:365–373.
7 Editorial: Microdialysis in human skin. Clin Exp Allergy 1995;25:1027–1029.
8 Petersen LJ, Stahl Skov P, Bindslev-Jensen C, Søndergaard J: Histamine release in immediate-type hypersensitivity reactions in intact human skin measured by microdialysis. Allergy 1992;47:635–637.
9 Petersen LJ, Kristensen JK, Bulow J: Microdialysis of the interstitial water space in human skin in vivo: Quantitative measurement of cutaneous glucose concentrations. J Invest Dermatol 1992; 99:357–360.
10 DeBoer J, Baarsma R, Okken A, Plijter-Groendijk H, Korf J: Application of transcutaneous microdialysis and continuous flow analysis for on-line glucose monitoring in newborn infants. J Lab Clin Med 1994;124:210–217.
11 Andersson T: Cutaneous microdialysis, a technique for human in vivo sampling. Linköping University Medical Dissertations No 456, 1995.
12 Andersson T, Svensson C, Anderson C: The effect of probe depth on histamine levels in human in vivo cutaneous microdialysis. Skin Res Technol 1996;in press.
13 Anderson C, Svensson C, Sjögren F, Andersson T, Wårdell K: Human in vivo microdialysis technique can be used to measure cytokines in contact reactions. Curr Probl Dermatol. Basel, Karger, 1995,Vol 23, pp 121–130.
14 Escher S, Schmelz M, Bickel A, Fartasch M, Diepgen T, Handwerker H: Quantification of plasma extravasation by dermal microdialysis in different types of inflammation (neurogenic versus non-neurogenic) (abstract). Allergologie 1995;18:464.
15 Anderson C, Andersson T, Molander M: Ethanol absorption across human skin measured by in vivo microdialysis technique. Acta Derm Venereol 1991;71:389–393.
16 Anderson C, Andersson T, Andersson RGG: In vivo microdialysis estimation of histamine in human skin. Skin Pharmacol 1992;5:177–183.
17 Anderson C, Andersson T, Wårdell K: Changes in skin circulation after insertion of a microdialysis probe visualized by laser Doppler perfusion imaging. J Invest Dermatol 1994;102:807–811.
18 Boman A, Wahlberg JE: Percutaneous absorption of three organic solvents in the guinea pig. I. Effects of physical and chemical injuries to the skin. Contact Dermatitis 1989;21:36–45.
19 Andersson T, Wårdell K, Anderson C: Human in vivo cutaneous microdialysis: Estimation of histamine release in cold urticaria. Acta Derm Venereol 1995;75:343–347.
20 Wahlberg JE: Percutaneous absorption. Curr Probl Dermatol. Basel, Karger, 1973, vol 5, pp 1–36.
21 Hegemann L, Forstinger C, Partsch B, Lagler I, Krotz S, Wolff K: Microdialysis in cutaneous pharmacology: Kinetic analysis of transdermally delivered nicotine. J Invest Dermatol 1995;104: 839–843.

Dr. Chris Anderson, Department of Dermatology, University Hospital,
S-581 85, Linköping (Sweden)

Elsner P, Lachapelle JM, Wahlberg JE, Maibach HI (eds): Prevention of Contact Dermatitis. Curr Probl Dermatol. Basel, Karger, 1996, vol 25, pp 47–56

Influence of Evaporation and Repeated Exposure on the Percutaneous Absorption of Organic Solvents

Anders Boman[a], *Howard I. Maibach*[b]

[a] Department of Occupational Dermatology, National Institute for Working Life, Solna, Sweden;
[b] Department of Dermatology, School of Medicine, University of California, San Francisco, Calif. USA

The organic solvents constitute a large heterogeneous group of structurally and physico-chemically different chemical compounds with a number of common properties that have made them useful in industry. The properties they share are: (1) fluidity at room temperature; (2) lipophilicity; (3) volatility with a varied rate of evaporation; (4) inexpensiveness; (5) systemic and local toxicity.

The fluidity and lipophilicity are the properties most commonly applied. Fluid solvents are used for dissolving of organic compounds, for instance in paints and glues, in degreasing applications and as intermediates in organic synthesis. The volatility of solvents is also used in vapor degreasing applications. Some solvents also have a substantial water solubility, making them useful for amphiphilic dissolution of such as in water-based paints. The toxicity of solvents ranges from inducing mild narcosis to lethality when absorbed systemically. Experimental data show that several of the solvents are lethal when the skin is exposed [1–3]. Most are also locally toxic following their skin exposure inducing necrosis, erythema, and edema [4–11]. A few solvents or their metabolites are sensitizers [12–16].

The physicochemical properties of solvents – volatility, molecular weight, lipophilicity, water solubility – vary substantially and are summarized for a few solvents in table 1. As can be seen these properties vary considerably.

Table 1. Physicochemcial properties of some organic solvents

Solvent	MW	Density	Vapor pressure, 25 °C mm Hg	Boiling point °C	Water solubility mg/100 ml	log $P_{Oct/W}$
Alcohols						
Methanol	32.04	0.7924	96.1	64.5	∞	–0.68
Ethanol	46.07	0.7937	44.0	78.3	∞	–0.31
Propanol	60.09	0.8050	14.5	97.2	∞	0.30
n-Butanol	74.12	0.8109	4.39	117.7	7,800	0.88
Polyhydric alcohols, glycols						
Ethylene glycol	62.07	1.1155	0.06	197.3	∞	–1.93
Propylene glycol	76.09	1.0381	0.05	187.4	∞	–
Aromatics						
Benzene	78.12	0.879	100	80.1	180	2.13
Toluene	92.15	0.8623	28.4	110.6	82	2.6
Styrene	104.14	0.9012	6.54	145.2	i.s.	2.95
Aliphatics						
Pentane	72.15	0.645	400	36.1	3.7	3.62
n-Hexane	86.17	0.660	100	68.7	i.s.	3.6
n-Heptane	100.19	0.684	40	98.4	0.3	4.66
Octane	114.22	0.703	10	125.7	0.07	5.18
Chlorinated aliphatics						
Chloroform	119.38	1.485	243	61.2	820	1.97
Trichloroethylene	131.39	1.455	56.0	86.7	100	2.29
Tetrachloroethylene	165.83	1.627	28	121.0	40	2.60
1,1,1-Trichloroethane	133.44	1.321	100	74.4	50	2.49
1,1-Dichloroethane	98.96	1.1680	304	57.3	–	1.79
1,2-Dichloroethane	98.96	1.255	64	83.6	0.870	1.48
Esters						
Ethyl acetate	88.11	0.9006	100	77.1	9,000	0.73
Butyl acetate	116.16	0.880	9.0	126.5	780	–
Ethers						
Methyl ether	46.07	0.661	3,982	–24.9	35,300	0.10
Ethyl ether	74.12	0.7146	442.0	34.5	6,900	0.83
Glycol ethers						
Methoxyethanol	76.10	0.9663	6	124.5	∞	–0.77
Ethoxyethanol	90.12	0.9311	4	135.6	∞	–0.54
Butoxyethanol	118.18	0.9019	0.6	171.2	∞	0.83

Table 1 (continued)

Solvent	MW	Density	Vapor pressure, 25 °C mm Hg	Boiling point °C	Water solubility mg/100 ml	log $P_{Oct/W}$
Ketones						
Acetone	58.05	0.792	400	56.1	∞	–0.24
Methyl ethyl ketone	72.11	0.806	75.6	79.6	80,600	0.29
Amides						
Dimethyl formamide	73.09	0.9445	3.7	153.0	∞	–1.01
Acetonitrile	41.05	0.7868	73	81.6	∞	–0.43
1-Methyl-2-pyrrolidone	99.13	1.0278	5.17	202	∞	–
Miscellaneous solvents						
Acrylonitrile	41.05	0.7857	73	81.6	∞	–0.34
Dimethyl sulfoxide	78.13	1.1014	0.47	189.0	∞	–1.35
Dioxane	88.1	1.0329	29.0	101.1	∞	–0.27
Limonene	136.23	0.8402	1.43	176.0	i.s.	–
Pyridine	79.10	0.978	20	115.2	∞	0.64
Turpentine	–	0.85–0.87	–	155–175	i.s.	–
White spirit	–	0.75–0.80	–	150–215	i.s.	–
Thinner	–	–	–	–	–	–
Petroleum ether	–	–	–	30–60	–	–

∞ = Completely miscible with water; i.s. = practically insoluble in water.

After skin exposure several chemicals show a substantial loss of compound from the skin surface, not only by absorption but also by evaporation [17–21]. The volatility of solvents is the prerequisite for their skin loss through evaporation, the major route of loss from the skin surface of these and other compounds with high vapor pressure.

Figure 1 summarizes the differing chemical structures of a few organic solvents. The purpose of the present investigation was to study the influence of repeated exposure on the in vivo percutaneous absorption of three organic solvents, and how ventilation influenced the in vitro percutaneous absorption of two of these solvents.

Materials and Methods

In vivo Exposure

Albino guinea pigs were anesthetized with sodium pentobarbital. A catheter was inserted into the jugular vein. The hair on the skin of the back was cut with electric clippers. A glass ring (Ø 2cm) was glued to the exposed area using a solvent-resistant glue (Cyanoacrylate). The depot so formed was filled with 0.5 ml neat solvent and exposure was open. In the continuous exposure it was left in the depot for 240 min. Intermittent exposure was for 1 min, each 30 min, whereafter the solvent was removed with a pipette and the skin gently wiped with cotton. To exclude respiratory exposure, the animals were given fresh air to their breathing zone, and exposure was carried out on a ventilated bench.

Blood (0.5 ml) was removed at regular intervals during the exposure. The blood loss was compensated for by injecting equal amounts of Macrodex (Pharmacia, Uppsala). The blood samples were collected in glass vials and sealed. The blood solvent concentration was analyzed with a head space technique using a method described in detail elsewhere [22].

In vitro Exposure

Human dermatomed skin was obtained at autopsy and stored frozen until used. The skin was thawed for 1 h, cut into pieces and mounted into all-glass absorption/evaporation cells (Laboratory Glass Apparatus, Berkeley, Calif., USA). The skin was allowed to acclimatize for 1 h prior to exposure. The perfusion fluid (saline or saline with 6% PEG20) was stirred and the flow was maintained at a rate sufficiently high to ensure sink conditions.

The solvents studied were ^{14}C-n-butanol and ^{14}C-toluene. 250 µl of tracer-marked solvent was put into each cell. Ventilation was generated by coupling the exhaust end of the ventilation tower to a vacuum pump, the airflow regulated by individual flowmeters. The flows studied were 0, 90, 400 and 900 ml/min. The perfusion fluid was collected hourly and subsequently counted with a scintillation counter.

Results

Figure 2 shows the absorption profiles of toluene and n-butanol for the in vivo continuous and intermittent exposures. There is a clear difference in blood levels between the continuous exposure and the intermittent exposure for both solvents studied, with a serrated pattern of the blood concentration during the intermittent exposure but an even increase in the continuous exposure. The intermittent exposure was significantly lower during the whole exposure. For butanol there was a tendency to increased absorption during the intermittent exposure.

A plot of the total amount of solvent absorbed in relation to its volatility shows a clear relationship between the amount absorbed and vapor pressure (fig 3).

The absorption profile of neat toluene over human skin under nonventilated and ventilated conditions in vitro is shown in figure 4. A steady state

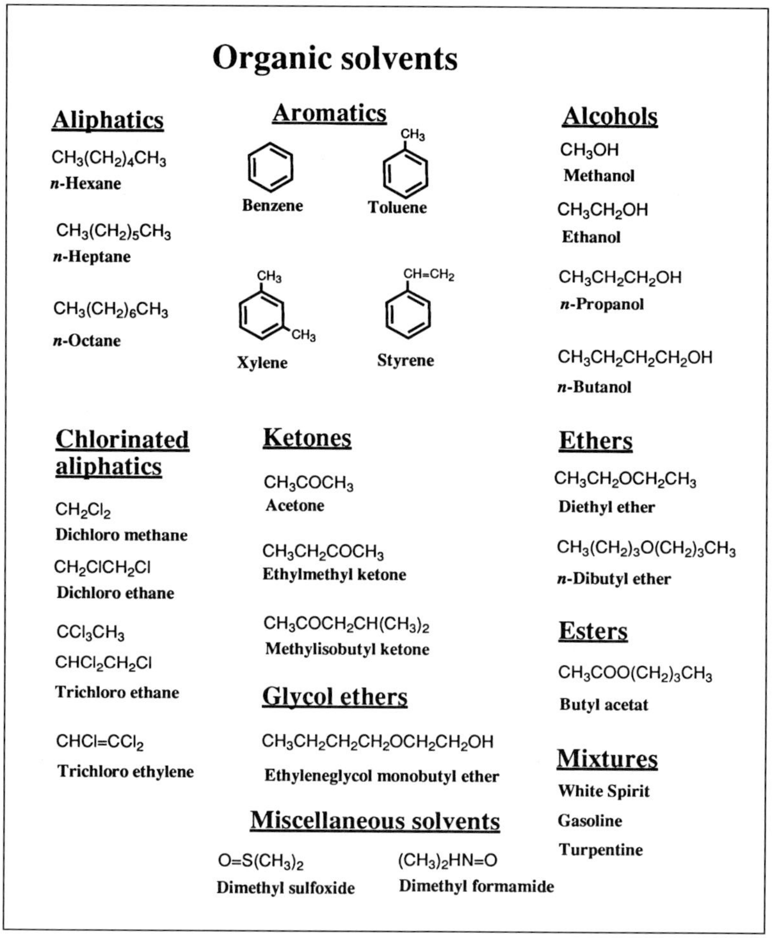

Fig. 1. Structural formulas of some organic solvents.

absorption is established at the nonventilated exposure after a few hours exposure. However, the ventilated exposure did not reach a steady state. The absorption profile of neat n-butanol over human skin under the same conditions as for toluene is shown in Figure 5. No steady state absorption was established neither for the ventilated exposure nor for the unventilated. A relationship between the absorbed dose and the speed of the ventilating airstream was noted for both solvents studied. The lowest ventilation rates generated the same initial absorption rates as the nonventilated exposure and then gradually decreased as the amount of solvent decreased. There was a clear tendency to lower absorption at higher ventilation rates. The total amount of

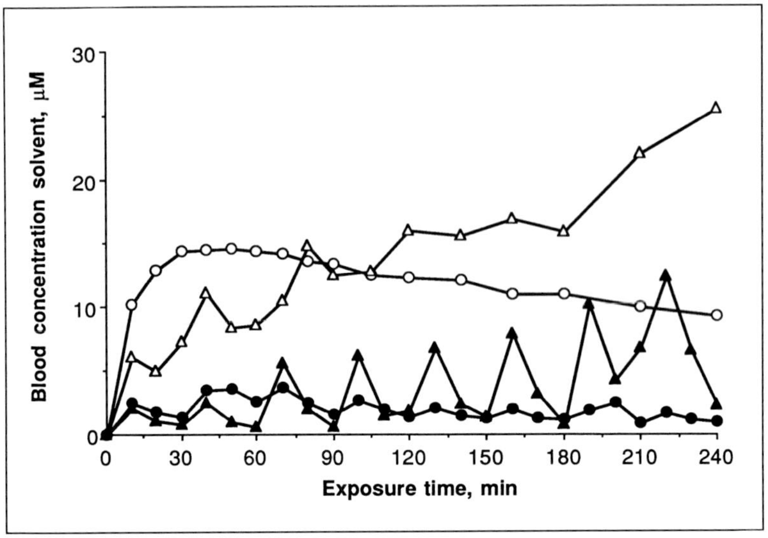

Fig. 2. Percutaneous absorption in guinea pigs in vivo of toluene and butanol during continuous and intermittent exposure. Toulene: continuous (○); intermittent (●); butanol: continuous (△); intermittent (▲).

Table 2. Influence of ventilation air flow rate on in vitro skin absorption of toluene and butanol

Air flow, ml/min	Absorbed dose, % of applied	
	toluene	butanol
90	0.77	1.09
400	0.53	0.70
900	0.17	0.25

solvent absorbed during the exposure time was related to the airflow rate (table 2). The solvent with the highest volatility toluene also gives the lowest amount absorbed.

Discussion

The interest in evaporative loss of compounds during skin exposure has mainly concentrated on insect repellents [17, 18]. Their evaporation from the skin surface is functionally important for the insect-repelling-process and a minimum effective dose can be established which is a balance of effect and duration of evaporation. However, in the major occupational environment,

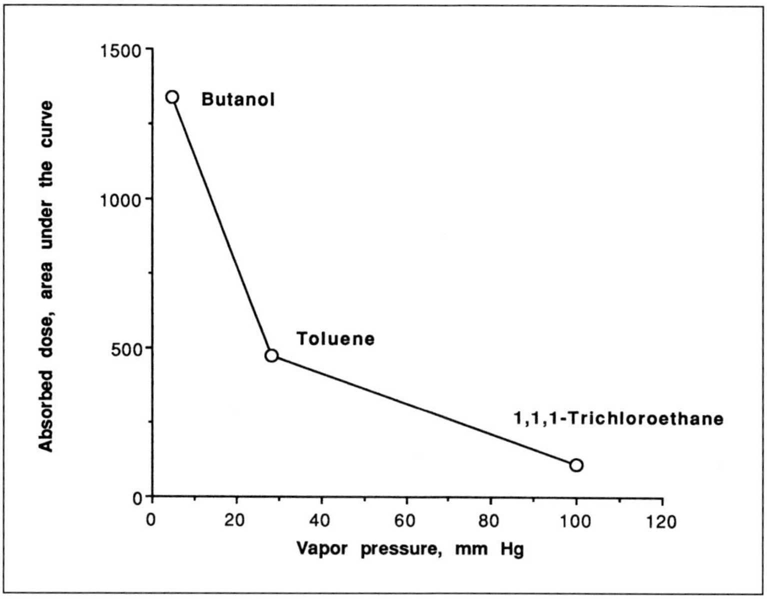

Fig. 3. Total percutaneous absorption (AUC) of toluene, 1,1,1,-trichloroethane and butanol during intermittent absorption.

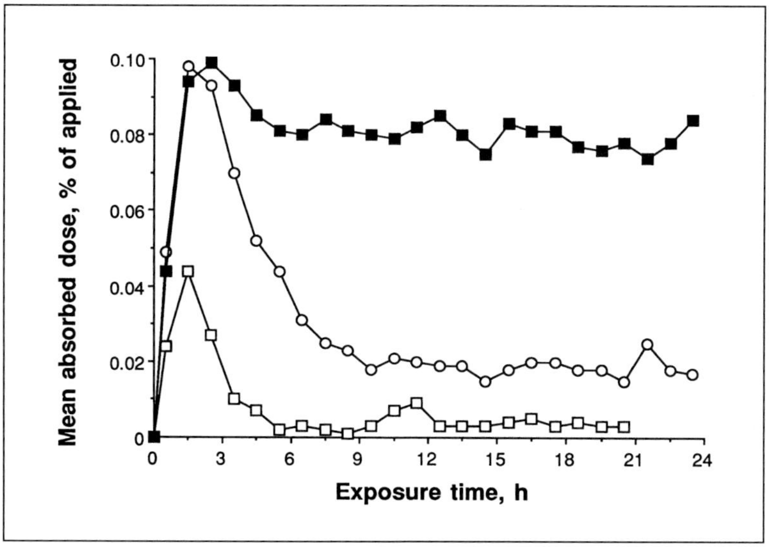

Fig. 4. In vitro percutaneous absorption of toluene in human skin during ventilation. Nonventilated exposure (■), ventilated 90ml/min (○), 900 ml/min (□).

evaporative loss of compound from the skin can be the major route of loss if an exposing compound has a sufficiently high vapor pressure. Little emphasis has been put on this aspect in occupational hygiene. Apart from the insect repellents, few occupationally important compounds have been studied in any depth. Occupational exposure is often brief and at variable intervals, which, unfortuantely does not favor the use of protective equipment. Unless gloves are put on from the start of a work shift, it often seems too much bother to use e.g. gloves only during critical exposure times, and thus the skin is exposed briefly at intervals.

Most organic solvents can be expected to show a substantial loss through evaporation on nonoccluded skin exposure, as they generally have a high vapor pressure (table 1). The observed difference in absorption profiles and absorbed amounts between the solvents studied in the intermittent in vivo exposure is most likely attributable to their differences in vapor pressure, and following evaporation. This is demonstrated in figure 3 by the almost linear relationship between the absorbed amount and the vapor pressure of the compounds studied. However, other mechanisms may contribute such as differences in toxicokinetics and distribution of the solvents at variable exposure and body concentrations. The influence of intermittent exposure on skin absorption of a volatile compound with a result confirming ours has been shown by Stewart and Dodd [23]. They found a considerably reduced absorption in humans at intermittent exposure to 1,1,1-trichloroethane compared to continuous exposure. Evaporative loss of chemicals with various vapor pressures has been discussed by Reifenrath and Spencer [21]. They studied the evaporative loss of various compounds and it ranged from a few percent for compounds with low vapor pressure to over 50% for those with the highest vapor pressures. Although the relationship was not linear the results agree with our results for the solvents studied.

As an evaporative loss of compound from an unoccluded skin surface can be expected particularly when the vapor pressure is high, well regulated ventilation at the working place may be of importance. To estimate this influence of ventilation rate on absorption through human skin of volatile solvents, we also studied this in an in vitro system. The results show that there was a clear relationship between the ventilation rate and the amount absorbed. The highest ventilation rate gave fast evaporation of the compound, which was seen as a rapid decrease in absorption. No steady state was reached during the ventilated exposures. The importance of ventilation rate has also been shown by Reifenrath and Spencer [21]. In the interval of ventilation rate they studied (30–60 ml/min), evaporation increased from 45 to 54% of applied dose and a concurrent reduction of amount absorbed. A result that corroborated ours and has implications for occupational hygiene.

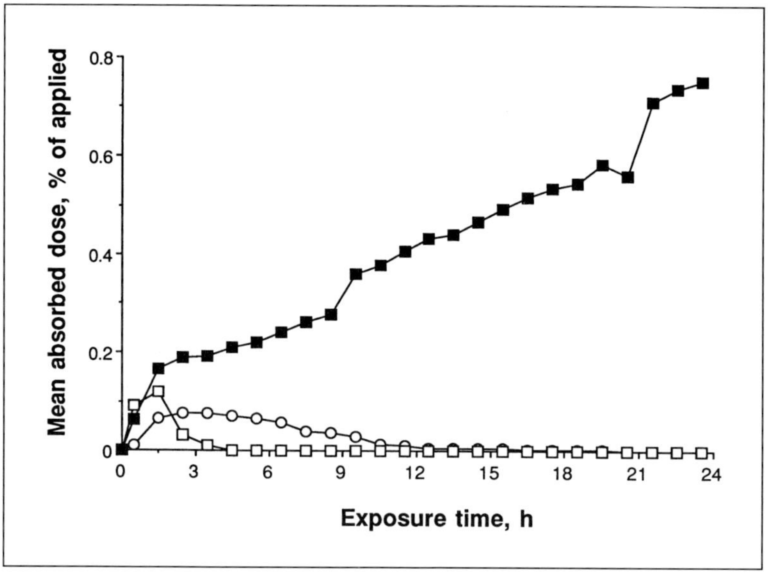

Fig. 5. In vitro percutaneous absorption of butanol in human skin during ventilation. Nonventilated exposure (■); ventilated 90 ml/min (○), 900 ml/min (□).

Conclusions

Based on the presented results, it is evident that in vivo skin absorption of volatile organic solvents at intermittent exposure is lower than under continuous conditions and the absorption is related to the volatility of the solvents. It was also demonstrated that the in vitro skin absorption with ventilation is related to the volatility of the solvent and also to the rate of ventilation. As a result of this, a sufficient workplace ventilation is an important occuptional hygienic measure not only to reduce exposure via respiration but also to reduce absorption of volatile compounds via the skin.

Acknowledgements

The technical assistance of the following persons is gratefully acknowledged: Gunnel Hagelthorn, Gunborg Lindahl, Kerstin Magnusson. The former Swedish work health fund provided the funds for the in vivo reasearch and a grant to A.B. as a visiting fellow at the UCSF. The Department of Dermatology, UCSF, is also gratefully acknowledged for making arrangements for A.B. as a visiting fellow.

References

1 Wahlberg JE: Percutaneous toxicity of solvents: A comparative investigation in the guinea pig with benzene, toluene and 1,1,2-trichloroethane. Ann Occup Hyg 1976;19:115–119.

2 Wahlberg JE, Boman A: 2-Chloroethanol: Percutaneous toxicity of a solvent. Dermatologica 1978; 156:299–302.

3 Wahlberg JE, Boman A: Comparative percutaneous toxicity of ten industrial solvents in the guinea pig. Scand J Work Environ Health 1979;5:345–351.

4 Wahlberg JE: Erythema-inducing effects of solvents following epicutaneous administration to man: Studied by laser Doppler flowmetry. Scand J Work Environ Health 1984;10:159–162.

5 Wahlberg JE: Assessment of erythema: A comparison between the naked eye and laser Doppler Flowmetry; in Frosch PJ, Dooms-Goosens A, Lachapelle J-M, Rycroft RJG, Scheper RJ (eds): Current Topics in Contact Dermatitis. Heidelberg, Springer, 1989, pp 549–553.

6 Wahlberg JE, Nilsson G: Skin irritancy from propylene glycol. Acta Derm Venereol 1984;64: 286–290.

7 Wahlberg JE: Propylene glycol: Search for a proper and nonirritant patch test preparation. Am J Contact Derm 1995;5:156–159.

8 Wahlberg JE: Edema-inducing effect of solvents following topical administration. Dermatosen 1984; 32:91–94.

9 Wahlberg JE: Measurement of skin-fold thickness in the guinea pig: Assessment of edema-forming capacity of cutting fluids, acids, alkalis, formalin, and dimethyl sulfoxide. Contact Dermatitis 1993; 28:141–145.

10 Kronevi T, Wahlberg JE, Holmberg B: Histopathology of skin, liver and kidney after epicutaneous administration of five industrial solvents to guinea pigs. Environ Res 1979;19:56–69.

11 Kronevi T, Wahlberg JE, Holmberg B: Skin pathology following epicutaneous exposure to seven organic solvents. Int J Tiss Reac 1981;3:21–30.

12 Pirilä V, Siltanen E: On the chemical structure of turpentine. Dermatologica 1958;117:1–8.

13 Fregert S, Håkanson R, Rorsman H, Tryding N, Övrum P: Dermatitis from alcohols: With special reference to possible impurities and metabolites. J Allergy 1963;5:404–408.

14 Sjöborg S, Dahlquist I, Fregert S, Trulson L: Contact allergy to styrene with cross reaction to vinyltoluene. Contact Dermatitis 1982;8:207–208.

15 Sjöborg S, Fregert S, Trulson L: Contact allergy to styrene and related chemicals. Contact Dermatitis 1984;10:94–96.

16 Karlberg A-T, Boman A, Melin B: Animal experiments on the allergenicity of *d*-limonene: The citrus solvent. Ann Occup Hyg 1991;35:419–426.

17 Spencer TS, Hill JA, Feldman RJ, Maibach HI: Evaporation of diethyltoluamide from human skin in vivo and in vitro. J Invest Dermatol 1979;72:317–319.

18 Reifenrath WG, Robinson PB: In vitro skin evaporation and penetration characteristics of moscito repellents. J Pharm Sci 1982;71:1014–1018.

19 Hawkins GS, Reifenrath WG: Development of an in vitro model for determining the fate of chemicals applied to the skin. Fund Appl Toxicol 1984;4:S133-144.

20 Hawkins GS, Reifenrath WG: Influence of skin source, penetration cell fluid, and partition coefficient on in vitro skin penetration. J Pharm Sci 1986;75:378–381.

21 Reifenrath WG, Spencer TS: Evaporation and penetration from human skin; in Bronaugh RL, Maibach HI (eds): Percutaneous absorption. Mechanisms – Methodology – Drug Delivery, ed 2. New York, Dekker, 1989, pp 313–334.

22 Boman A, Wahlberg JE: Percutaneous absorption of 3 organic solvents in the guinea pig, I. Effect of physical and chemical injury to the skin. Contact Dermatitis 1989;21:36–45.

23 Stewart RD, Dodd HC: Absorption of carbon tetrachloride, trichloroethylene, tetrachloroethylene, methylene chloride, and 1,1,1-trichloroethane through human skin. Ind Hyg J 1964;25:439–446.

Dr. Anders Boman, National Institute for Working Life, S–171 84 Solna (Sweden)

Elsner P, Lachapelle JM, Wahlberg JE, Maibach HI (eds): Prevention of
Contact Dermatitis. Curr Probl Dermatol. Basel, Karger, 1996, vol 25, pp 57–66

Prevention of Contact Dermatitis from Solvents

Jan E. Wahlberg, Anders Boman

Department of Occupational Dermatology, Karolinska Hospital Stockholm and
National Institute for Working Life, Solna, Sweden

Skin exposure to solvents can cause different types of adverse effects, as summarized in table 1. Most common is the irritant contact dermatitis seen in painters, mechanics and industrial workers. Allergic contact dermatitis from solvent is today a rare event, but was previously seen in painters and others exposed to turpentine [1]. Scleroderma is also rare and it is not clear from the literature whether the main route of exposure is percutaneous or by inhalation [2]. Local toxic reactions have been described experimentally [3, 4].

Percutaneous Absorption and Systemic Toxicity of Solvents

To be able to perform their action in the deeper strata of the skin, solvents have to be able to penetrate the skin barriers. The percutaneous absorption of several organic solvents has been studied with various techniques, in vitro and in vivo, using a variety of species – human as well as animal models (table 2). This absorption is regulated mainly by the concentration gradient across the skin, but other factors may also contribute [5–7]. Several of the industrial solvents have notations for skin absorption in the different occupational hygiene standards. However, there is still scant information on most solvents regarding their absorption rates, permeability coefficients and lag times for absorption through human skin; data that may be of great value in risk assessment. Future information is also needed on how various factors influence this absorption. In most cases statements on the behavior of solvents are based on inference from results with other

Table 1. Side effects of organic solvents at skin exposure

Irritancy/contact urticaria
Irritant contact dermatitis
Allergic contact dermatitis
Scleroderma
Percutaneous absorption – systemic toxicity

Table 2. Percutaneous absorption, toxicity and TLV skin notations of organic solvents

Solvent	Skin absorption data available			Skin toxicity	Systemic toxicity at skin exposure (2ml) in guinea pigs	TLV skin notation			Ref.
	J	Kp	other			USA	FRG	Sweden	
n-Hexane	–	–	×	×	nonlethal	–	–	–	3, 9
n-Butylacetate	–	–	–	×	–	–	–	–	3
Ethanol	×	×	–	–	–	–	–	–	14
n-Butanol	×	×	×	×	–	×	–	×	7, 14
2-Chloroethanol	–	–	–	×	lethal	×	×	×	3, 17, 18
2-Butoxyethanol	×	×	–	–	lethal	×	×	×	10, 11, 13, 14, 18
Methyl ethyl ketone	×	–	–	–	–	–	–	–	14
Methyl iso-butyl ketone	×	×	–	–	–	–	–	–	12
Benzene	×	–	×	×	nonlethal	–	×	×	4, 9, 14, 16, 18
Styrene	×	–	–	–	–	–	–	×	14
Toluene	×	×	×	×	nonlethal	–	–	×	3, 6, 9, 14, 16, 18
Carbon tetrachloride	×	–	×	×	lethal	–	×	×	3, 9, 18
1,2-Dibromoethane	–	–	×	×	–	–	×	–	4, 9
1,2-Dichloroethane	×	–	×	×	–	–	–	×	4, 9, 14
1,1,2,2-Tetrachloroethane	×	–	×	×	–	×	×	–	4, 9, 14
Tetrachloroethylene	×	–	×	×	–	–	–	–	4, 9, 14
1,1,1-Trichloroethane	×	–	×	×	nonlethal	–	–	–	4, 5, 9, 14
1,1,2-Trichloroethane	–	–	×	×	lethal	×	×	–	8, 16, 18
Trichloroethylene	–	–	×	×	nonlethal	–	–	–	4, 9, 14, 18
Dimethylformamide	×	–	–	–	lethal	×	×	×	14, 18

J = Data on permeability flux available; Kp = data on permeability coefficient available.

chemicals although these may differ considerably in physicochemical properties from solvents [6–14].

The systemic effect of solvents after skin absorption may be severe and fatalities in man have been reported [15]. Experimental studies show a great variability of the systemic effects of solvents in skin exposure [16–18]. Where solvents with high absorption rates and/or systemic toxicity are handled, the use of adequate skin protection is mandatory.

Prevention by Selection

Already in 1947, Klauder and Brill [19] stated that irritant action like defatting decreases as the boiling increases. By using the noninvasive laser Doppler technique, it was demonstrated that common solvents differ greatly in their irritant potential. This technique is 3–4 times more sensitive than the naked eye [20–23]. As shown in table 3, the most potent solvents were dimethyl sulfoxide and trichloroethylene, where 1 min of skin exposure was sufficient to affect skin blood flow. On the other hand, methyl ethyl ketone, propylene glycol and ethanol did not influence skin blood flow (15 min exposure, in excess, neat) [20–30]. Methyl ethyl ketone and ethanol are recommended as vehicles when patch testing with materials brought by patients. The whitening seen after rubbing skin, contaminated with solvent, is probably due to an effect on skin lipids rather than on skin blood flow [20, 24].

Edema caused by skin exposure to solvents can be quantified with a rather unsophisticated device – the caliper [25, 26]. Results from measurements of skin fold thickness in experimental animals and skin blood flow measurements in man are summarized in table 4. The ranking based on these three parameters can be used in the selection process when looking for solvents with absent or minimal skin-irritating properties for use in industry, laboratory work, etc. This must, however, be balanced against technical requirements such as dissolvability and TLVs.

Selection Based on Individual Susceptibility and Counseling

Individuals with a history of, or with current, atopic dermatitis are considered to be more susceptible to various irritants, including solvents (table 5). This knowledge should be used at preemployment examination and in vocational counseling. Concerning individuals with asthma and/or rhinitis, but not atopic dermatitis, it is not settled whether they also should be advised to avoid occupations involving exposure to solvents.

Table 3. Duration of skin exposure to solvents in excess (1.5 ml/3.1 cm^2) required to cause an increase in skin blood flow, objectively recorded with laser Doppler flowmetry in man

Exposure time	Solvents
1 min	dimethylsulfoxide trichloroethylene
5 min	n-hexane carbon tetrachloride 1,1,1-trichloroethane 1,1,2-trichloroethane 1,4-diethylbenzene
15 min	dodecane
>15 min no effect	methyl ethyl ketone propylene glycol ethanol[1] water

[1] Slight decrease.

Table 4. Ranking of erythema- and edema-inducing effects of solvents

Solvents	Erythema skin blood flow laser Doppler flowmetry in man	Edema skinfold thickness	
		rabbit	guinea pig
Trichloroethylene	1	1	1
Dimethyl sulfoxide	2	2	2
n-Hexane	3	4	5
Carbon tetrachloride	3	2	4
Toluene	4	1	2
1,1,1-Trichloroethane	5	2	4
Ethanol	–	6	6
Propylene glycol	–	3	6
Methyl ethyl ketone	–	3	6

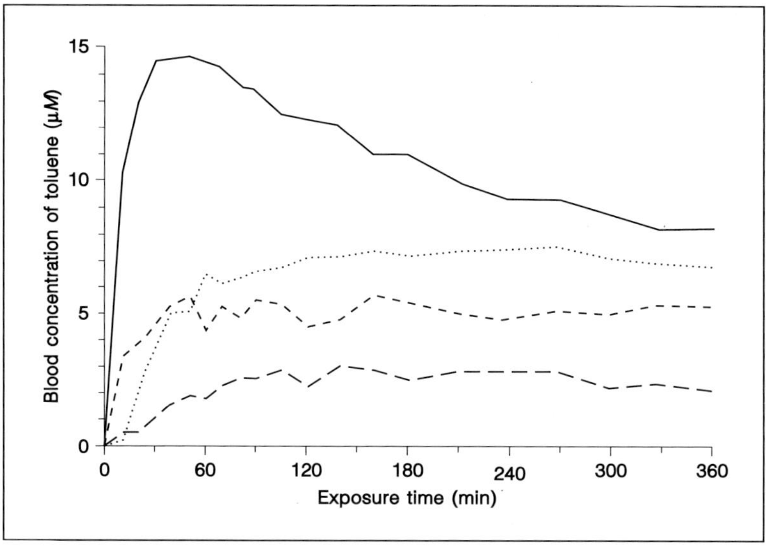

Fig. 1. Percutaneous absorption in vivo in guinea pigs of toluene during exposure with and without glove protection. Neat solvent on unprotected skin (———) and on skin protected with PVC (··········), butyl rubber (– – – – –), and natural rubber (- - - - - - -) gloves. After Boman and Mellström [41].

Table 5. Individual susceptibility to organic solvents

Considerable variation
Predisposition/increased susceptibility to solvents in individuals with a history of atopic dermatitis
History of asthma/rhinitis: not settled
Individuals with a history of contact dermatitis
Pre-employment examination

Table 6. Conclusions

Reduce exposure
Appropriate selection – great variation in potency (irritancy, percutaneous absorption, toxicity)
Gloves – some protection
Barrier creams – still matter for debate
Individual susceptibility
Skin care program
Legislation, labeling, information

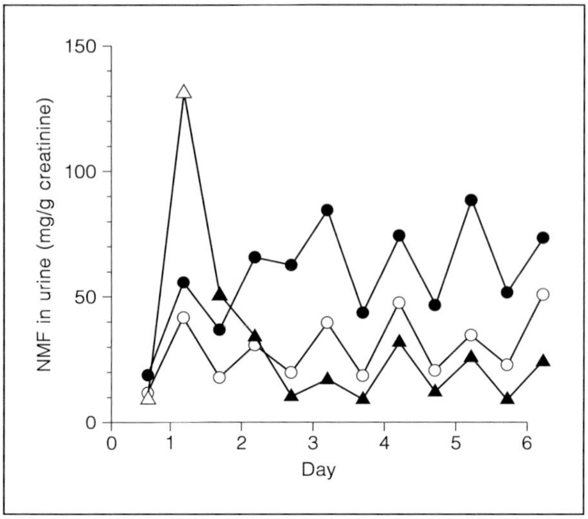

Fig. 2. Effect of protective equipment on uptake of dimethyl formamide during work. Pre- and postshift excretion of N-methylformamide during barrier cream (—●—), gloves (—○—), and respiratory protection 1st day (—△—) followed by skin protection (—▲—). Redrawn from Lauwerys et al. [46].

Protective Effects of Gloves and Barrier Creams

As the hands and forearms are the sites where most irritant dermatitis occurs, protection of these areas from exposure is of utmost importance. The most obvious and best prophylactic measure is to strictly avoid any skin contact with the noxious chemical or replace the noxious chemical by one with a less adverse effect. However, this is not always possible for technical reasons and management must provide means for proper skin protection for the workers. Protective equipment available on the market comprises protective gloves of polymeric materials, and barrier creams. The efficacy of barrier creams is dealt with in a separate chapter in this volume and will only be mentioned briefly [27]. Several studies have shown barrier creams to have some protective effect against the acute irritative and locally toxic actions of solvents [28, 29]. However, for more extended exposure times they do not seem to be effective [30, 31]. The barrier properties against systemic absorption are also less than adequate [32–35].

Protective gloves, if selected according to recommendations, may provide a protection which allows for work in direct contact with solvents for several hours [36–38]. The basis for these recommendations is data gathered in tech-

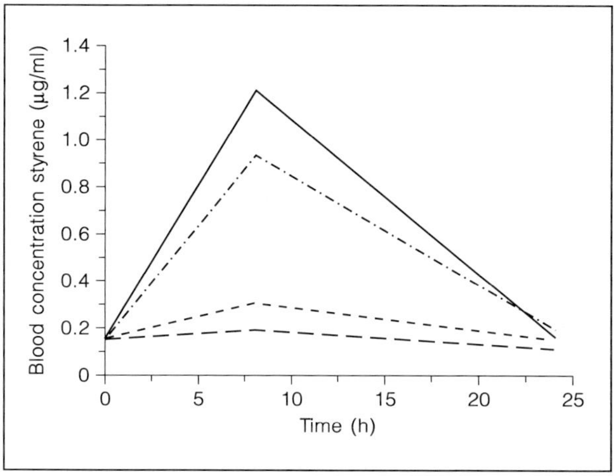

Fig. 3. Effect of protective means on absorption of styrene during work. Blood concentration of styrene during unprotected work (——), protective clothes (–·—·), work with respiratory protection (–––), respiratory protection and protective clothes (— — —). After Brooks et al. [47].

nical testing or in vivo studies. The technical testing is well standardized and described in CEN and ASTM standards [39, 40]. The in vivo testing is performed in various ways, ranging from ordinary patch testing to animal exposure (fig. 1) and work site studies [41–45].

A classic study is the one performed by Lauwerys et al. [46] in an acrylic fibre mill. The varying efficacy of barrier creams and gloves and the importance to use proper skin protection at work with a solvent with low vapor pressure and high skin absorption conditions is clearly demonstrated for dimethyl formamide (fig. 2). Workers were followed for 3 weeks. During the first week gloves were used as skin protection, which resulted in some absorption of DMF. During the second week a glycerol-based barrier cream was used and this was less protective than the gloves and the caution to avoid skin exposure.

The efficacy of various protective equipments in exposure to styrene, a solvent with physiocochemical properties different from those of DMF, was investigated by Brooks et al. [47]. In this case, absorption is mainly through inhalation. Respiratory protection (a mask) was crucial and the additional protection of gloves was minor (fig 3).

Conclusions

Based on information found in the literature and on our own experience, recommendations for reducing skin side effects of exposure to solvents are summarized in table 6. Quantitative data on skin irritant properties (table 4) and percutaneous absorption and toxicity (table 2) are good starting points for the selection process. The wearing of gloves will obviously temporarily reduce skin exposure to solvents, but today's gloves are still not perfect and more reliable ones are highly desirable [36]. The protective effect of barrier creams in skin exposure is still an open question.

References

1 Rudzki E, Berova N, Czernielewski A, Grzywa Z, Hegyi E, Jiràsek J, Kalensky J, Michailov P, Nebenführer A, Rothe A, Schubert H, Stransky L, Szarmach H, Temesvári E, Ziegler V: Contact allergy to oil of turpentine: A 10-year retrospective view. Contact Dermatitis 1991;24:317–318.

2 Czirják L, Pócs E, Szegedi G: Localized scleroderma after exposure to organic solvents. Dermatology 1994;189:339–401.

3 Kronevi T, Wahlberg JE, Holmberg B: Histopathology of skin, liver and kidney after epicutaneous administration of five industrial solvents to guinea pigs. Environ Res 1979;19:56–69.

4 Kronevi T, Wahlberg JE, Holmberg B: Skin pathology following epicutaneous exposure to seven organic solvents. Int J Tiss Reac 1981;3:21–30.

5 Wahlberg JE: Skin permeability and disorders. Scand J Work Environ Health 1985;11(suppl 1): 96–97.

6 Boman A, Wahlberg JE: Percutaneous absorption of 3 organic solovents in the guinea pig. (I). Effect of physical and chemical injury to the skin. Contact Dermatitis 1989;21:36–45.

7 Boman A: Factors influencing the percutaneous absorption of organic solvents: An experimental study in the guinea pig. Arbete och Hälsa 1989;11.

8 Jacobson I, Holmberg B, Wahlberg JE: Variations in the blood concentration of 1,1,2-trichloroethane by percutaneous absorption and other routes of administration in the guinea pig. Acta Pharmacol Toxicol 1977;41:497–506.

9 Jacobson I, Wahlberg JE, Holmberg B, Johansson G: Uptake via the blood and elimination of 10 organic solvents following epicutaneous exposure of anaesthetized guinea pigs. Toxicol Appl Pharmacol 1982;63:181–187.

10 Johansson G, Fernström P: Percutaneous uptake rate of 2-butoxyethanol in the guinea pig. Scand J Work Environ Health 1986;12:499–503.

11 Johansson G, Boman A, Dynésius B: Percutaneous absorption of 2-butoxyethanol in man. Scand J Work Environ Health 1988;14:101–109.

12 Wigaus-Hjelm E, Boman A, Fernström P, Hagberg M, Johanson G: Percutaneous uptake and kinetics of methyl isobutyl keytone (MIBK) in the guinea pig. Toxicol Lett 1991;56:79–86.

13 Johanson G, Boman A: Percutaneous absorption of 2-butoxyethanol vapour in human subjects. Br J Ind Med 1991;48:788–792.

14 Grandjean P: Skin Penetration: Hazardous Chemicals at Work. London, Taylor & Francis, 1990.

15 Lington AW, Bevan C: Alcohols; in Clayton GD, Clayton FE (eds): Patty's Industrial Toxicology ed 4. New York, Wiley, 1994, pp 2731–2735.

16 Wahlberg JE: Percutaneous toxicity of solvents: A comparative investigation in the guinea pig with benzene, toluene and 1,1,2-trichloroethane. Ann Occup Hyg 1976;19:115–119.

17 Wahlberg JE, Boman A: 2-Chloroethanol: Percutaneous toxicity of a solvent. Dermatologica 1978; 156:299–302.

18 Wahlberg JE, Boman A: Comparative percutaneous toxicity of ten industrial solvents in the guinea pig. Scand J Work Environ Health 1979;5:345–351.
19 Klauder JV, Brill FA: Correlation of boiling ranges of some petroleum solvents with irritant action on the skin. Arch Derm Syph 1947;56:197–215.
20 Wahlberg JE: Erythema-inducing effects of solvents following epicutaneous administration to man: Studied by laser Doppler flowmetry. Scand J Work Environ Health 1984;10:159–162.
21 Wahlberg JE: Assessment of erythema: A comparison between the naked eye and laser Doppler flowmetry; in Frosch PJ, Dooms-Goossens A, Lachapelle J-M, Rycroft RJG, Scheper RJ (eds): Current Topics in Contact Dermatitis. Heidelberg, Springer, 1989, pp 549–553.
22 Wahlberg JE, Nilsson G: Skin irritancy from propylene glycol. Acta Derm Venereol 1984;64:286–290.
23 Wahlberg JE: Propylene glycol: Search for a proper and nonirritant patch test preparation. Am J Contact Derm 1995;5:156–159.
24 Goldsmith LB, Friberg SE, Wahlberg JE: The effect of solvent extraction on the lipids of the stratum corneum in relation to observed immediate whitening of the skin. Contact Dermatitis 1988;19: 348–350.
25 Wahlberg JE: Edema-inducing effect of solvents following topical administration. Dermatosen 1984; 32:91–94.
26 Wahlberg JE: Measurement of skin-fold thickness in the guinea pig: Assessment of edema-forming capacity of cutting fluids, acids, alkalis, formalin, and dimethyl sulfoxide. Contact Dermatitis 1993; 28:141–145.
27 Lachapelle J-M: Efficacy of protective creams; in Elsner P, Lachapelle J-M, Wahlberg JE, Maibach HI, (eds): Prevention of Contact Dermatitis. Curr Probl Dermatol. Basel, Karger, 1996;25:182–192.
28 Mahmoud G, Lachapelle JM, van Neste D: Histological assessment of skin damage by irritants: Its possible use in the evaluation of a 'barrier cream'. Contact Dermatitis 1984;11:179–185.
29 Mahmoud G: Evaluation of the protective value of an antisovent gel by laser Doppler flowmetry and histology. Contact Dermatitis 1985;13:14–19.
30 Frosch PJ, Kurte A: Efficacy of skin barrier creams. I. The repetitive irritation test (RIT) in the guinea pig. Contact Dermatitis 1993;28:94–100.
31 Frosch PJ, Kurte A: Efficacy of skin barrier creams. IV. The repetitive irritation test (RIT) with a set of 4 standard irritants. Contact Dermatitis 1994;31:161–168.
32 Lauwerys RR, Dath T, Lachapelle J-M, Buchet J-P, Roels H: The influence of two barrier creams on the percutaneous absorption of m-xylene in man. J Occup Med 1978;20:17–20.
33 Boman A, Wahlberg JE, Johansson G: A method for the study of the effect of barrier creams and protective gloves on the percutaneous absorption of solvents. Dermatolgica 1982;164:157–160.
34 Boman A, Mellström G, Wahlberg JE: Protective effect of barrier creams against skin absorption of organic solvents in guinea pigs; in Mellström G, Carlsson B (eds): Second Scandinavian Symposium on Protective Clothing Against Chemicals and Other Health Risks. Solna Arbetslivsinstitutet, Arbete och Hälsa 1987, vol 12, pp 12–19.
35 Boman A, Mellström G: Percutaneous absorption of 3 organic solvents in the guinea pig. III. Effect of barrier creams. Contact Dermatitis 1989;21:134–140.
36 Mellström GA, Wahlberg JE, Maibach HI: Protective Gloves for Occupational Use. Boca Raton, CRC Press, 1994.
37 Mellström GA, Boman AS: Gloves: Types, materials and manufacturing; in Mellström GA, Wahlberg JE, Maibach JE, Maibach HI (eds): Protective Gloves For Occupational Use. Boca Raton, CRC Press, 1994, pp 21–35.
38 Mellström G, Boman A, Wahlberg JE: Protective gloves. Reduction of skin exposure to chemicals; in Maibach HI (ed): Occupational and Industrial Dermatology, ed 2. Chicago, Year Book, 1987, pp 126–133.
39 Mellström GA, Landersjö L, Boman AS: Permeation of neoprene protective gloves by acetone: Comparison of three different permeation cells in an open-loop system. Am Ind Hyg Assoc J 1989; 50:554–559.
40 Mellström GA, Carlson B, Boman AS: Testing of protective effect against liquid chemicals; in Mellström GA, Wahlberg JE, Maibach HI (eds): Protective Gloves For Occupational Use. Boca Raton, CRC Press, 1994, pp 53–57.

41 Boman A. Mellström G: Percutaneous absorption of 3 organic solvents in the guinea pig. IV. Effect of protective gloves. Contact Dermatitis 1989;21:260–266.

42 Boman A, Wahlberg JE: Bioassay for the testing of protective glove performance against skin absorption of organic solvents; in Barker RL, Coletta GC (eds): Performance of Protective Clothing. Philadelphia, ASTM, 1986, STP 900, pp 214–220.

43 Boman A, Wahlberg JE: In vivo assessment of synthetic barriers against percutaneous absorption of organic solvents in the guinea pig; in Maibach HI, Lowe NJ (eds): Models in Dermatology. Basel, Karger, 1989, vol 4, pp 193–201.

44 Mellström G, Boman A: Comparative evaluation of permeation testing of protective gloves to solvent: In vitro permeation cells versus in vivo in guinea pigs. Contact Dermatitis 1992;26:120–127.

45 Boman AS, Mellström GA: Percutaneous absorption studies in animals; in Mellström GA, Wahlberg JE, Maibach HI (eds): Protective Gloves for Occupational Use. Boca Raton, CRC Press, 1994, pp 91–107.

46 Lauwerys RR, Kivits A, Lhoir M, Rigolet, P, Houbeau D, Buchet J-P, Roels H: Biological surveillance of workers exposed to dimethylformamide and the influence of skin protection on its percutaneous absorption. Int Arch Occup Environ Health 1980;45:189–203.

47 Brooks SM, Anderson L, Emmett E, Carlson A, Tsay J-Y, Elia V, Buncher R, Karbowsky R: The effects of protective equipment on styrene exposure in workers in the reinforced plastics industry. Arch Environ Health 1980;35:287–294.

Prof. Jan E. Wahlberg, National Institute for Working Life, S–171 84 Solna (Sweden)

Elsner P, Lachapelle JM, Wahlberg JE, Maibach HI (eds): Prevention of Contact Dermatitis. Curr Probl Dermatol. Basel, Karger, 1996, vol 25, pp 67–77

An Immunohistochemical Study on Mild Skin Irritation Induced by a Single Application of a Low-Molarity Sodium Dodecyl Sulfate Solution: Keys to the Prevention of Irritant Contact Dermatitis

Mai Le, Simone Cals, Joost Schalkwijk, Pieter van der Valk

Department of Dermatology, University Hospital Nijmegen, The Netherland

Chronic irritant contact dermatitis (CICD) is considered to be caused by repeated exposure of the skin to irritant effects of various nature [1]. It is often characterized by hyperkeratotic or dyskeratotic, fissured, slightly erythematous, slowly spreading patches [2]. In contrast to acute irritant reactions, the tendency to heal is small. Decrease in contact with the irritants does not always lead to healing.

Repeated exposure to weak irritants may lead to adaptation, repair or disease. The skin reacts with an inflammatory response and with concomitant changes in epidermal growth.

Willis et al. [3] demonstrated cytopathic effects on keratinocytes (dyskeratosis and parakeratosis) and a strong inflammatory response, hallmarked with a large number of neutrophils after a 48-hour exposure of 5% (w/v) SDS. Recently, we found changes in epidermal growth including upregulation of cycling cells, involucrin, and epidermal fatty acid binding protein (E-FABP) after a 4-hour exposure time of 5% (w/v) SDS. We observed a mild inflammation characterized by the absence of polymorphonuclear leukocytes (PMNs), but with a mild mononuclear perivascular infiltrate [4]. A shorter exposure time as compared to the study of Willis et al. [3] may account for the difference in inflammatory response.

Multiple factors such as the characteristics of the irritant, exposure time, additional irritant effects and environmental conditions, make it difficult to study skin irritation by chemicals and consequently makes it difficult to study the pathogenesis of CICD. To understand the mechanisms underlying the pathogenesis we need experimental models. Many investigators use sodium dodecyl sulfate (SDS) as a standard irritant in their models [5–8].

A model must mimic the daily exposure to irritant effects as well as possible. Therefore, a model with repeated application of a mild irritant is needed. A mild irritant which induces no macroscopical cutaneous reaction after one but induces macroscopical and microscopical skin changes after multiple exposures. To find an appropriate exposure model low concentrations of SDS were used in a pilot study. We pipetted 200 μl of a dilution series of SDS (w/v) (5, 1, 0.2 and 0.04%) on patches [4] and exposed the skin to these patches during 4 h. Cutaneous reaction (as judged by erythema) and transepidermal water loss (TEWL) were assessed after removal of the patches. In this pilot study, we found that 0.2% SDS solution induced a small but significant increase in TEWL compared to normal skin, whereas no erythema was observed. The concentrations 1 and 5% caused mild-to-intense erythema and TEWL increased significantly. SDS 0.04% (w/v) did not increase TEWL significantly and did not elicit erythema in the subjects tested.

In the present study we have studied inflammation and changes in epidermal proliferation and differentiation after a single application of low concentrations (0.2 and 1%) of SDS to find the most appropriate concentration. Using the monoclonal antibody, MIB-1, which can direct to the Ki-67 antigen present in the proliferating cells, a polyclonal antibody to SKALP/elafin, a protein associated with inflammatory/hyperproliferative conditions [9–11], and MON-150, an antibody to involucrin, a cytoplasmic protein precursor of cornified envelope [12–14], we studied changes in epidermal growth. In addition we studied the inflammatory response in HE sections.

Materials and Methods

Subjects

A total of 17 healthy volunteers (10 males and 7 females) took part in this study, ranging in age from 20 to 28 years (mean age 25 years).

Patch Testing

We used a 1% and a 0.2% dilution of SDS (w/v). The application, exposure and sampling procedure was identical to the procedure described in a previous study [4]. Briefly, an aliquot of 200 μl of SDS was pipetted on a patch, consisting of a 1.5-cm^2 piece of absorbent, nonwoven fabric on a 4.0-cm^2 piece of impermeable plastic foil. All subjects were patch tested on the back for 4 h.

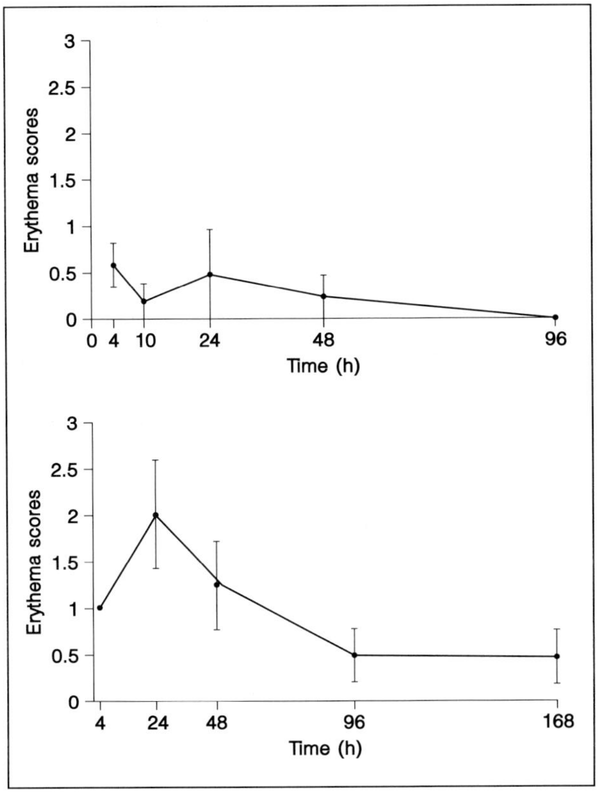

Fig. 1. The time course of mean erythema scores after application of 0.2% SDS (top) and 1% SDS (bottom).

Clinical Assessment and Transepidermal Water Loss (TEWL) Measurements

After removal of the patches, we graded erythema. TEWL was measured at timepoints: 0, 4, 10, 24, 48 and 96 h for 0.2% SDS and at 0, 4, 24, 48, 96 and 168 h (day 7) for 1% SDS. Visual scores were assigned to each patch test reaction according to the following scale: 0 = no visible reaction; 1 = faint, patchy erythema; 2 = diffuse mild erythema; 3 = moderate erythema; 4 = intense erythema. TEWL measurements were done using a Tewameter TM 210 (Courage & Khazaka, Germany) according to standard guidelines [15].

Staining Procedures

Immunohistochemical stainings were performed on 6-mm paraffin sections of a total of 46 punch biopsies (3 mm diameter) with the MIB-1 antibody, with a polyclonal antibody to SKALP/elafin and with MON-150 according to standard procedures, described in a previous study [4]. The monoclonal antibody MIB-1 recognizes the proliferation-associated Ki-67 antigen on formalin fixed material (Immnunotech. S.A., Marseille, France). The polyclonal antibody directed against recombinant SKALP/elafin and the monoclonal antibody MON-150 directed against human involucrin were prepared and characterized as we previously described [16, 17]. HE staining was done according to Mayer.

Histological Examination

The number of proliferative keratinocytes was assigned by counting the number of MIB-1-positive nuclei per mm length of section. The involucrin expression was quantified by assessing the number of positively staining layers on two representative areas (supra- and interpapillary) of the epidermis. The ratio of positive layers and the total number of cell layers was calculated.

Statistical Methods

Student's t test was used for statistical analysis.

Results

Visual Grading and TEWL Measurements

No erythema was observed at any time point after 0.2% SDS application. Exposure to 1% SDS induced patchy mild erythema to diffuse mild erythema and gave a maximum at 24 h (fig. 1). Following the 0.2% SDS exposure, a small increase in TEWL was measured. The TEWL after treatment with 1% SDS was higher as compared to normal skin and reached a maximum on day 2. Figure 2 shows the time course of TEWL of both concentrations of SDS.

Histological Findings

HE Staining. Sections after treatment of both concentrations, 0.2 and 1%, of SDS showed neither parakeratosis nor apparent spongiosis. No obvious edema in the papillary dermis was seen. A very mild perivascular infiltrate consisting of mononuclear cells was observed in most sections. In general, the morphology of skin treated with 0.2 or 1% SDS hardly differed from that of normal skin.

Epidermal Proliferation. In normal untreated skin the number of MIB-1 positively staining cells is 56 ± 8 (mean $\pm$ SEM) per mm length of section. Following application of 0.2% SDS no significant increase in the number of MIB-1-positive cells was shown in comparison with normal skin. In contrast, a marked increase of the MIB-1-positive cells was observed after exposure to 1% SDS. The maximum of 176 ± 48 (mean $\pm$ SEM) was reached at day 2 after stimulation, whereas the number of proliferating cells of normal skin amounted to 56 ± 17 (mean $\pm$ SEM). At day 7 the number of MIB-1-positive cells had not reached the baseline. Figure 3 illustrates the number of the MIB-1-positive cells after exposure to the two concentrations of SDS.

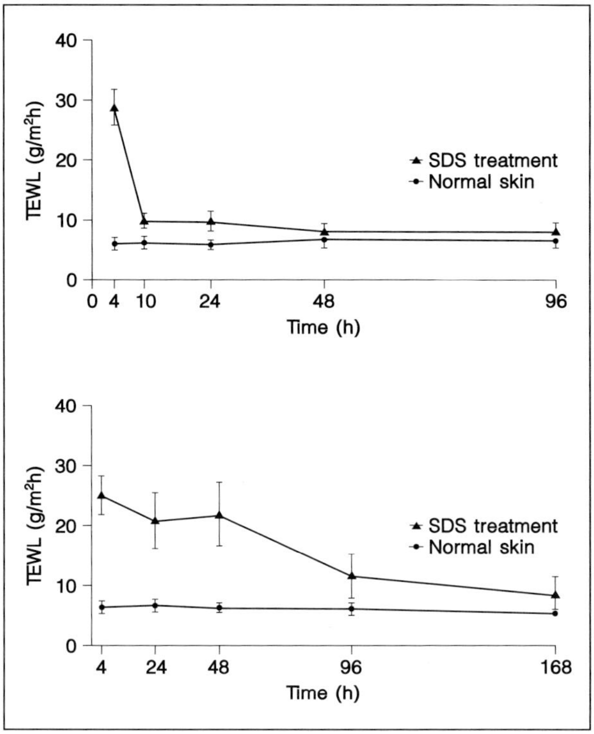

Fig. 2. The time course of TEWL following 0.2% SDS (top) and 1% SDS (bottom).

Epidermal Differentiation. SKAPL/elafin, a molecule known as an epidermal hyperproliferation/inflammation marker, was expressed in 1–2 layers of the stratum granulosum at 24 h after application of both concentrations. Surprisingly, no induction of SKALP/elafin was found at any other time point. Quantitative assessment of the MON-150-positive cell layers in the epidermis suggested that there was little or no difference between irritant-treated and normal skin following 0.2% SDS application. In contrast, a strong upregulation of involucrin was observed which peaked at day 2 after 1% SDS application (fig. 4). At day 7 after stimulation the expression of involucrin had reached the normal value.

Figure 5 illustrates the immunohistochemical findings.

Correlation between TEWL, Erythema, Number of Cycling Cells and Involucrin Expression

We correlated data on TEWL, erythema scores, number of the MIB-1-positive cells and the percentage of the MON-150-positive epidermal cell layers

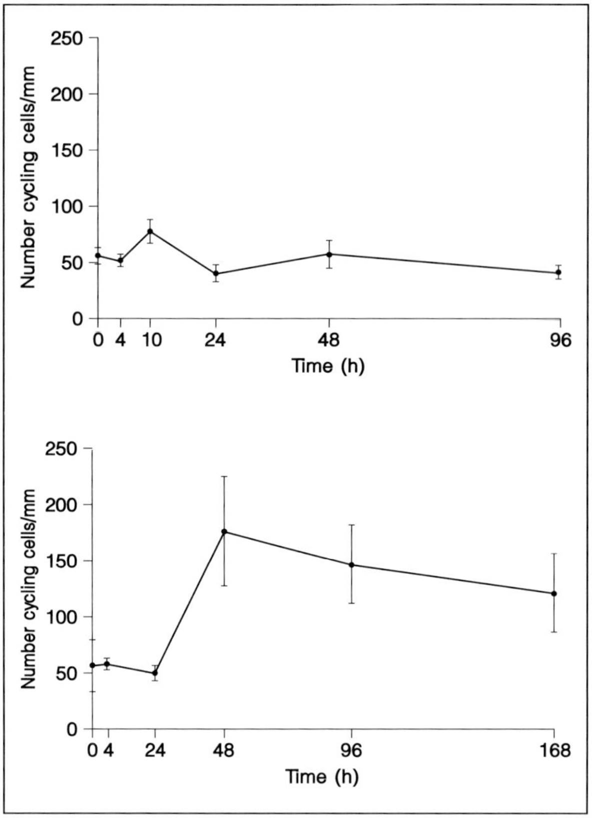

Fig. 3. The kinetics of MIB-1-positive nuclei, representing the rate of basal cell division in the epidermis after 0.2% SDS (top) and 1% SDS (bottom). The values are calculated from number of cycling cells per mm length of section (mean ± SEM).

obtained at day 2 following the application of 0.2, 1 [this study] and 5% of our previous study [4]. In table 1 the correlation coefficients (r) and level of significance (p values) are summarized.

Discussion

Repeated exposure of the skin to various irritant effects may lead to adaptation, repair or disease. If the skin can cope with intensity and frequency of the stimuli, the horny layers become thicker, no skin disease will be observed. When damaging effects are stronger and last longer beyond a certain limit,

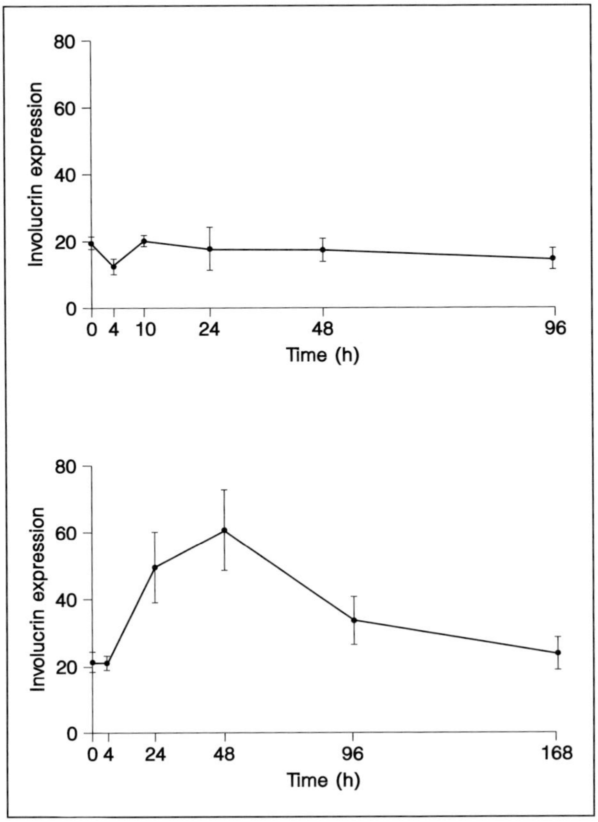

Fig. 4. Expression of involucrin (MON-150-stained cell layers) within 4 days after 0.2% SDS (top) and within 7 days after 1% SDS (bottom). The values are expressed as a percentage of the total of epidermal cell layers (mean ± SEM).

irritant contact dermatitis can occur [1]. Adaptation makes the skin less and disease more vulnerable to irritants. A small damage to a diseased skin can sustain irritant contact dermatitis. Therefore, limiting the exposure to irritant effects is more successful in the prevention of irritant contact dermatitis than healing in diseased skin.

Chemicals can have a direct influence on the stratum corneum but may also cause a secondary inflammatory response after damaging the viable layers of the epidermis [18]. These secondary effects can also result in alteration in formation and function of stratum corneum. After a single exposure to a mild irritant the skin can control the inflammation and the barrier function will be repaired. Cumulative exposure to irritants, however, may lead to CICD. It

Table 1. The correlation between four parameters: erythema scores, TEWL, MIB-1 and involucrin

Parameters	Correlation coefficient (r)	Significance (p)
TEWL vs. erythema	0.91	0, $3.3 \cdot 10^{-5}$
TEWL vs. MIB-1	0.77	0.004
TEWL vs. involucrin	0.79	0.002
Erythema vs. MIB-1	0.75	0.005
Erythema vs. involucrin	0.74	0.006
MIB-1 vs. involucrin	0.88	0.0001

Pooled data obtained from day 2 after treatment of 0.2, 1 and 5% SDS (n = 12).

is unclear why the process can become chronic and why healing does not or occurs slowly.

We suggest that changes in the epidermal proliferation and differentiation play at least additionally a role in the chronicity of the disease.

Compounds influencing epidermal growth may be useful in treating CICD. Corticosteroids have been used in the treatment of many inflammatory skin diseases because of their potent anti-inflammatory effects [19]. Topical corticosteroids, however, can cause atrophy and may make the skin more vulnerable to irritants. Whether topical corticosteroids substantially modulate skin irritation is in debate [20, 21]. Using TEWL and visual scoring, we found that neither the topical corticosteroids nor the vehicle inhibited visible response to the irritant significantly [22]. The use of topical corticosteroids in CICD is in our view limited.

Previous studies have shown that administering retinoids can inhibit the formation of the cornified envelope in cultured human keratinocytes [23, 24]. Topical or systemic treatment with retinoids may modulate epidermal growth. The retinoids now available are however restricted in their use because of skin irritation [25].

Various studies have demonstrated that the topical application of vitamin D_3 derivates (calcitriol and tacalcitol) can interfere with inflammation, epidermal proliferation and differentiation processes in psoriatic skin [26, 27]. Like retinoids vitamin D_3 derivates can, however, cause skin irritation [28]. Modulating early changes in inflammation, epidermal growth by topical or systemic treatment with new vitamin A or vitamin D_3 derivates, without skin irritant properties, may be candidates for healing CICD.

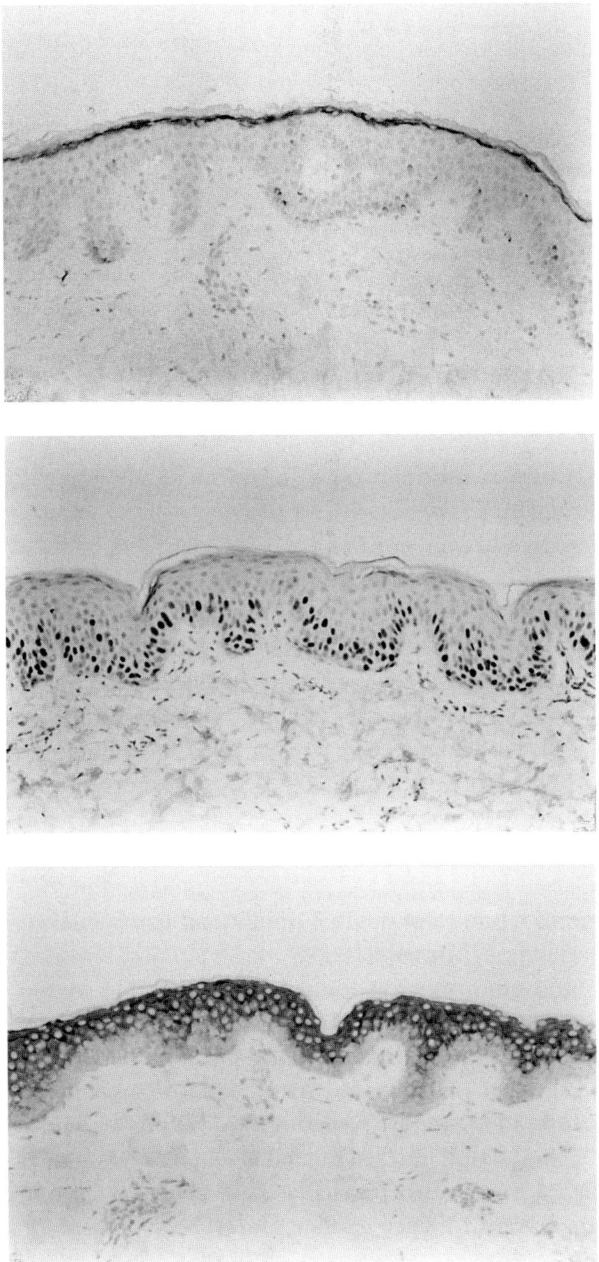

a

b

c

Fig. 5. Sections showing immunohistochemical staining of SKALP (top) 24 h after challenge with 0.2% SDS; MIB-1 (center) 48 h after stimulation with 1% SDS and involucrin (bottom) 48 h after challenge with 1% SDS.

We present a model in which the inflammatory response and concomitant changes in epidermal growth of the skin can be studied after a single application of 0.2% (w/v) SDS during 4 h. This model is considered to be appropriate for studying skin irritation by chemicals and consequently the pathogenesis of irritant contact dermatitis. Application of 0.2% SDS induced a small but significant increase in TEWL and no visible cutaneous reaction whereas no significant expression of SKALP/elafin was seen. Other immunohistochemical findings as MIB-1 and involucrin expression showed no difference between normal skin and skin treated with 0.2% SDS.

An immunohistochemical approach in this model in which the skin is repeatedly exposed to this low concentration SDS may provide insight into processes either leading to adaptation and repair or to disease. It may help to understand the mechanism underlying the pathogenesis of CICD which may also provide keys to prevention.

References

1 Malten KE: Thoughts on irritant contact dermatitis. Contact Dermatitis 1981;7:238–247.

2 Frosch PJ: Cutaneous irritation; in Rycroft RJG, Menne T, Frosch PJ (eds): Textbook of Contact Dermatitis, 2. Berlin, Springer, 1995, pp 28–61.

3 Willis CM, Stephens CJ, Wilkinson JD: Differential patterns of epidermal leukocyte infiltration in patch test reactions to structurally unrelated chemical irritants. J Invest Dermatol 1993;101: 364–370.

4 Le M, Schalkwijk J, Siegenthaler G, van de Kerkhof PCM, van der Valk PGM: Changes in keratinocyte differentiation following mild irritation by sodium dodecyl sulphate. 1996; in press.

5 van der Valk PG, Nater JP, Bleumink E: The influence of low concentrations of irritants on skin barrier function as determined by water vapour loss. Derm Beruf Umwelt Arch Dermatol Res. 1986, in press.

6 van der Valk PG, Nater JP, Bleumink E: Vulnerability of the skin to surfactants in different groups of eczema patients and controls as measured by water vapour loss. Clin Exp Dermatol 1985;10: 98–103.

7 Frodin T, Helander P, Molin L, Skogh M: Hydration of human stratum corneum studied in vivo by optothermal infrared spectrometry, electrical capacitance measurement, and evaporimetry. Acta Derm Venereol 1988;68:461–467.

8 Wilhelm KP, Freitag G, Wolff HH: Surfactant-induced skin irritation and skin repair. Evaluation of the acute human irritation model by noninvasive techniques. J Am Acad Dermatol 1994;30: 944–949.

9 Schalkwijk J, van Vlijmen IM, Alkemade JA, de Jongh GJ: Immunohistochemical localization of SKALP/elafin in psoriatic epidermis. J Invest Dermatol 1993;100:390–393.

10 Alkemade JA, Molhuizen HO, Ponec M, Kempenaar JA, Zeeuwen PL, de Jongh GJ, van Vlijmen Willems IM, van Erp PE, van de Kerkhof PC, Schalkwijk J: SKALP/elafin is an inducible proteinase inhibitor in human epidermal keratinocytes. J Cell Sci 1994;107:2335–2342.

11 Wiedow O, Schroder JM, Gregory H, Young JA, Christophers E: Elafin: an elastase-specific inhibitor of human skin. Purification, characterization, and complete amino acid sequence (published erratum appears in J Biol Chem 1991;266:3356). J Biol Chem 1990;265:14791–14795.

12 Michel S, Schmidt R, Shroot B, Reichert U: Morphological and biochemical characterization of the cornified envelopes from human epidermal keratinocytes of different origin. J Invest Dermatol 1988;91:11–15.

13 Hohl D: Cornified cell envelope. Dermatologica 1990;180:201–211.

14 Watt FM: Terminal differentiation of epidermal keratinocytes. Curr Opin Cell Biol 1989;1:1107–1115.

15 Pinnagoda J, Tupker RA, Agner T, Serup J: Guidelines for transepidermal water loss (TEWL) measurement. A report from the Standardization Group of the European Society of Contact Dermatitis. Contact Dermatitis 1990;22:164–178.

16 Molhuizen HO, Alkemade HA, Zeeuwen PL, de Jongh GJ, Wieringa B, Schalkwijk J: SKALP/elafin: An elastase inhibitor from cultured human keratinocytes. Purification, cDNA sequence, and evidence for transglutaminase cross-linking. J Biol Chem 1993;268:12028–12032.

17 van Duijnhoven JL, Schalkwijk J, Kranenborg MH, van Vlijmen Willems IM, Groeneveld A, van Erp PE, Timmer ED, de Jongh GJ, van de Ven WJ: MON-150, a versatile monoclonal antibody against involucrin: Characterization and applications. Arch Dermatol Res 1992;284:167–172.

18 Berardesca E, Distante F: The modulation of skin irritation. Contact Dermatitis 1994;31:281–287.

19 Snell ES: The pharmacological properties of corticosteroids in relation to clinical efficacy. Br J Dermatol 1976;94(suppl 12):15–23.

20 Ramsing DW, Agner T: Efficacy of topical corticosteroids on irritant skin reactions. Contact Dermatitis 1995;32:293–297.

21 Berardesca E, Distante F, Vignoli GP, Rabbiosi G: Acute irritant dermatitis: Effect of short-term topical corticoid treatment; in Surber C, Elsner P, Bircher AJ (eds): Exogenous Dermatology: Advances in Skin-Related Allergology, Bioengineering, Pharmacology, and Toxicology, ed 1. Basel, Karger, 1995, vol 22, pp 86–90.

22 van der Valk PGM, Maibach HI: Do topical corticosteroids modulate skin irritation in human beings? Assessment by transepidermal water loss and visual scoring. J Am Acad Dermtol 1989;21:519–522.

23 Green H, Watt FM: Regulation by vitamin A of envelope cross-linking in cultured keratinocytes derived from different human epithelia. Mol Cell Biol 1982;2:1115–1117.

24 Fuche E, Green H: Regulation of terminal differentiation of cultured human keratinocytes by vitamin A. Cell 1981;25:617–625.

25 Boyd-AS: An overview of the retinoids. Am J Med 1989;86:568–574.

26 Gerritsen MJP, Rulo HFC, van Vlijmen-Willems I, van Erp PEJ, van de Kerkhof PCM: Topical treatment of psoriatic plaques with 1,25-dihydroxyvitamin D_3: A cell biological study. Br J Dermatol 1993;128:666–673.

27 Gerritsen MJP, Boezeman JBM, van Vlijmen-Willems IMJJ, van de Kerkhof PCM: The effect of tacalcitol (1,24 $(OH)_2D_3$) on cutaneous inflammation, epidermal proliferation and keratinization in psoriasis, a placebo-controlled, double-blind study. Br J Dermatol 1994;131:57–63.

28 Kragballe K, Steijlen PM, Ibsen HH, van de Kerkhof PC, Esmann J, Sorensen LH, Axelsen MB: Efficacy, tolerability, and safety of calcipotriol ointment in disorders of keratinization. Results of a randomized, double-blind, vehicle-controlled, right/left comparative study. Arch Dermatol 1995;131:556–560.

P.G.M. van der Valk, MD, PO Box 9101, NL–6500 HB Nijmegen (The Netherlands)

Elsner P, Lachapelle JM, Wahlberg JE, Maibach HI (eds): Prevention of Contact Dermatitis. Curr Probl Dermatol. Basel, Karger, 1996, vol 25, pp 78–85

Prevention of Surfactant-Induced Irritant Contact Dermatitis

Klaus-P. Wilhelm

proDERM Institute for Applied Dermatological Research, Schenefeld/Hamburg, Germany

It is undisputed that surfactants (detergents) play a dominant role as causative agents in the induction of chronic irritant contact dermatitis (ICD) [1–3]. ICD is not only a difficult skin disease to treat but produces significant disability in the workplace and to the citizen at large [4, 5]. Therefore, prevention of surfactant-induced ICD should be given more attention than therapy.

Surfactants

Surfactants (*surf*ace *act*ive *agents*) have – as the name implies – a modifying effect on the boundary surface between two immiscible phases, where one phase is usually liquid and the other is gas, usually air.

Soap had been the only available surfactant until the beginning of this century. Soap has been used for over 4,500 years as a general-purpose cleansing agent as well as for the treatment of wounds. *Syn*thetic *det*ergents (syndets) were first produced at the beginning of this century. Initially, syndets were used solely as laundry detergents. However, since the late 1940s, synthetic detergents have been used in increasingly growing proportions in personal washing products. Today's worldwide production of surfactants exceeds 20 million tons of which anionic surfactants account for over 50% [6].

Surfactant molecules possess both a relatively long nonpolar, hydrophobic part (tail) and a relatively small polar part (head). As an example, the molecular structure of the anionic surfactant sodium lauryl sulfate which is greatly used as a modul irritant is drawn in figure 1. This molecular structure is responsible for the micelle formation of surfactants and hence their ability to disperse

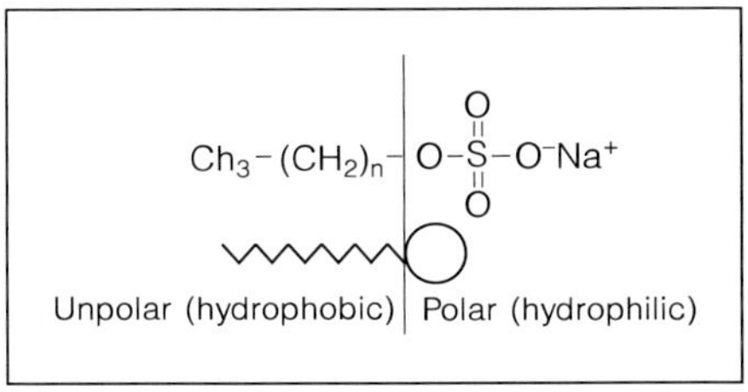

Fig. 1. Molecular structure of the model irritant sodium lauryl sulfate (SLS).

Table 1. Detergents/surfactants: classification according to hydrophilic group

Anionic surfactants
Alkyl sulfates
Alkyl sulfanates
Isothionates
Cationic surfactants
Alkyl quarternary ammonium compounds
Amphoteric surfactants
Betaines
Nanionic surfactants
Alkyl polyethoxylates

water-insoluble substances in an aqueous phase. The aggregation of surfactants on the surface boundary is responsible for the reduction of the surface tension and the induction of foam. These biophysical properties explain their cleansing, emulsfying and bactericidal activity which make them indispensible in a vast number of cosmetic and pharmaceutical products, e.g. shampoos, shower gels, toothpastes, creams.

Surfactants are somewhat arbitrarily classified according to the charge of their polar groups, into four classes (table 1). A complete review of available surfactants, their biophysical properties and application is beyond the scope of this article. For a review, see Falbe [7].

Surfactant-Induced Skin Irritation

The biophysical effects that determine the detergent properties of surfactants (table 2) are responsible for their irritation potential. The problem of soap irritation was already recognized in the 1930s by Blank [8]. Soap and

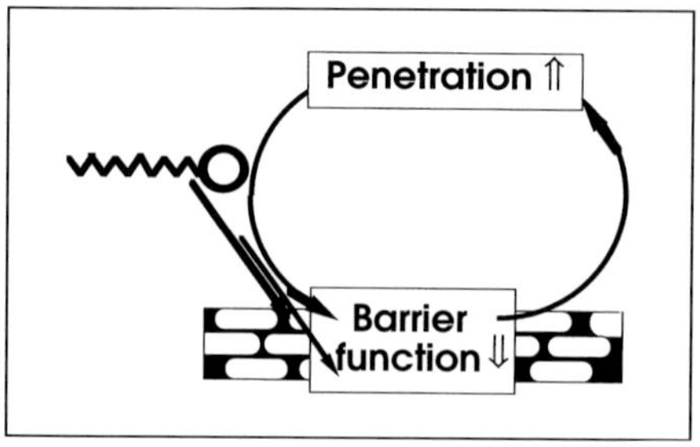

Fig. 2. Influence of surfactants on stratum corneum barrier function.

Table 2. Biophysical effects of surfactants

Disperse water-insoluble substances
Reduce tension between interfaces
Induce foam
Cleansing activity
Emulsifying activity
Bactericidal activity

Table 3. Pathophysiology of surfactant-induced ICD

Denaturation of SC proteins
Reorganization (extraction) of intercellular lipids
Decrease corneocyte cohesion
Impair skin barrier function
Increase TEWL
Enhance percutaneous penetration
Decrease SC water-binding capacity

synthetic surfactants exert a number of effects on the skin (table 3), especially the stratum corneum of which the temporary increase in skin surface pH induced by soap and alkaline surfactant products appears, contrary to the long-held belief, to be the least significant. The irritant effects of surfactants have been reviewed recently [3, 9].

The single most important effect of surfactants, especially anionic surfactants, is a perturbation of skin barrier function leading to increased percutaneous penetration of other chemicals applied to the skin as well as to an increased penetration of their own (fig. 2).

Table 4. Intolerance reactions against soaps/syndets

Authors, year	%	n
FDA study (1975)	12.6	589
Br. Consumers Assoc. (1979)	12.0	626
US Dept. of Commerce (1978)	9.5	698
Romaguera et al. (1983)	4.1	210
US Dept. of Commerce (1975)	3.7	8,399
Ngangu et al. (1983)	0	96

Cited from Ring and Gollhausen [14].

Detergent-induced ICD is therefore a self-aggravating disease. Moreover, chronic irritant dermatitis will often persist for years even if exposure to any irritant is minimized as far as possible. Various epidemiologic studies have demonstrated that even a job change does not always solve the problem [4, 10].

The barrier disruption which itself is invisible as well as the visible signs of surfactant-stratum corneum interaction, i.e. dryness, roughness and scaliness, are mainly due to a binding of surfactants to SC keratins with concomitant protein denaturation [11, 12] Insertion of surfactants into the intercellular lipid bilayers results in a fluidization of the lipoidal material and an additional increase in skin permeability whereas a removal of stratum corneum lipids has only been reported for exaggeratedly high concentrations and appears therefore to be of less relevance [13]. Unfortunately, most of our experimental knowledge about detergent-induced ICD is based on the exposure of skin to just one surfactant and this single substance has been in the vast majority of cases the nonionic surfactant SLS [3].

With the exception of certain amphoteric surfactants, e.g. cocamido propyl betaine and a few nonionic surfactants, e.g. propylene glycol, which reportedly are contact sensitizers, allergic contact dermatitis is rarely induced by surfactants [14]. While there is ample clinical and experimental evidence for the skin-irritating effects of surfactants no exact figures are available for incidence and prevalence rates for surfactant-induced ICD. Hence, intolerance reactions against soaps and syndets are reported to range from 0 to 12.6% (table 4).

However, there is no exposure to neat surfactants in real life because surfactant products contain additional constituents, i.e. perfumes, antioxidants, deodorants, dyes, refatting agents [7, 15]. Moreover, most products contain surfactant mixtures rather than only one surfactant. Therefore, it is often difficult to make the judgement that an irritant dermatitis in a given

Table 5. Prevention of detergent-induced ICD

Primary prevention
Elimination of damaging effects before induction of diseases
Secondary prevention
Diagnosis and therapy of diseases at an early stage
Tertiary prevention
Therapy of active diseases in order to prevent aggravations and complications

patient is truly caused by surfactant exposure. Most of the times the patients with irritant dermatitis have exposed their hands to a number of potentically irritant substances which in fact is almost impossible to avoid considering that even water has a potentially irritant capacity.

Humans will react quite differently to the same irritant stimulus. We have shown some years ago that some individuals will respond with lower skin irritation after exposure to 3% SDS than other individuals that are exposed to 0.1% SDS [16]. More recently we have demonstrated that these striking interindividual differences in the irritant susceptibility within the same ethnic group are indeed more pronounced than interethnic differences, e.g. between Germans and Chinese [17]. Therefore, it is more than justified to assume a multifactorial genesis of this disease.

Prevention of Surfactant-Induced ICD

As for any other disease three levels of prevention of surfactant-induced ICD can be discerned (table 5). The primary prevention, i.e. the elimination of offending/damaging effects will yield the most effective results and should therefore be the primary goal (table 6). However, the total elimination of the responsible agent is neither realistic nor desirable. The primary prevention of detergent-induced ICD would therefore consist of a reduction of contact between surfactants and the skin which can be achieved at the workplace by the introduction of 'no contact' automization processes and wearing of protective gloves (the latter aspect is covered elsewhere in this book). The replacement of surfactants with high irritation potential by substances with improved skin compatibility is another important step in the primary prevention of surfactant-induced skin irritation [18].

Table 6. Primary prevention of detergent-induced ICD

Reduce contact time
Gloves
Automization
Increase workers' (consumers') risk awareness
Replace (potential) irritants
Classify substances for their irritation potential
Develop detergents with better skin compatibility
Requires classification of potential irritants!

Table 7. Predictive tests in humans

Exaggerated exposure
Patch test
Single vs. repeated
Open vs. occluded
Immersion test
Exaggerated wash test
Use test
Field studies
Objective evaluation (bioengineering techniques) increases validity of predictive tests.

This process, however, requires a reliable classification of the irritation potential of all surfactants. The most relevant data are obtained by predictive skin tolerability studies in human volunteers [19–21]. However, a great number of different study protocols are available for this purpose (table 7) and a careful selection of the test procedure is highly recommended in order to obtain meaningful results.

Conclusions

As for most diseases – detergent-induced ICD is no exception – effective prevention can only be achieved by a multilevel, interdisciplinary effort. In contrast to many other diseases neither the extinction of the causative agents nor the total prevention of the contact between skin and detergents appear realistic in the foreseeable future.

Additionally complicating in the prevention of surfactant-induced ICD is the direct link between the wanted (surfactant properties) and unwanted (skin irritating effect) parts of these substances.

A realistic strategy for the prevention of detergent-induced ICD would therefore be to:

(1) minimize exposure;

(2) classify detergents according to their irritation potential;

(3) develop detergents (mixtures) with improved benefit-risk ratio;

(4) prevent disease at an early stage (use of barrier creams and moisturizers).

References

1 Tupker RA: The influence of detergents on the human skin; thesis, State University Groningen. The Netherlands, 1990.

2 van der Valk PJM, Nater JP, Bleumink E: Skin irritancy of surfactants as assessed by water vapor loss measurements. J Invest Dermatol 1984;82:291.

3 Effendi I, Maibach HI: Surfactants and experimental irritant contact dermatitis. Contact Dermatitis 1995;33:217–225.

4 Andersen KE, Benezra C, Burrows D, Camorasa J, Dooms-Goossens A. Ducombs G, et al: Contact dermatitis: A review. Contact Dermatitis 1987;16:55–78.

5 Mathias CGT, Morrison JH: Occupational skin diseases, United States: Results from the Bureau of Labor Statistics annual survey of occupational injuries and illnesses, 1973 through 1984. Arch Dermatol 1988;124:1519–1524.

6 Ainsworth SJ: Soaps and detergents. Chem Eng News 1992;70:27–63.

7 Falbe J: Surfactants in Consumer Products. Heidelberg, Springer, 1986.

8 Blank IH: Action of soap on skin. Arch Dermatol Syph 1939;39:811–824.

9 Frosch PJ: Irritancy of soaps and detergent bars in Frost P, Horwitz SN (eds): Principles of Cosmetics for the Dermatologist. St. Louis, Mosby, 1982, pp 5–12.

10 Rystedt I; Hand eczema and long-term prognosis in atopic dermatitis. Acta Derm Venereol 1985; (suppl 117):1–59.

11 Imokawa G, Sumura K, Katsumi M: Study on skin roughness caused by surfactants. II. Correlation between protein denaturation and skin roughness. J Am Oil Chem Soc 1975;52:484.

12 Wilhelm KP, Cua AB, Wolff HH, Maibach HI: Surfactant-induced stratum corneum hydration in vivo: Prediction of the irritation potential of anionic surfactants. J Invest Dermatol 1993;101: 310–315.

13 Imokawa G, Akasaki S, Minematsu Y, Kawai M: Importance of intercellular lipids in water-retention properties of the stratum corneum: Induction and recovery study of surfactant dry skin. Arch Dermatol Res 1989;281:45.

14 Ring J, Gollhausen R: Allergologische Bewertung von Syndets zur Hautreinigung; in Braun-Falco O, Korting HC (eds): Hautreinigung mit Syndets. Berlin, Springer, 1990, pp 181–188.

15 Jungermann E: The formulation and properties of syndet bars. Cosmet Toiletries 1982;97: 77–80.

16 Wilhelm KP, Surber C, Maibach HI: Quantification of sodium lauryl sulfate irritant dermatitis in man: Comparison of four techniques: Skin color reflectance, transepidermal water loss, laser Doppler flow measurement and visual scores. Arch Dermatol Res 1989;281:293.

17 Basketter DA, Griffiths HA, Wang XM, Wilhelm KP, McFadden J: Individual, ethnic and seasonal variability in irritant susceptibility of skin: The implications for a predictive human patch test. Contact Dermatitis 1996; in press.
18 Rhein LD, Simion FA, Hill RL, Cogan RH, Mattai J, Maibach HI: Human cutaneous response to a mixed surfactant system: Role of solution phenomena in controlling surfactant irritation. Dematologica 1990;180:18–23.
19 Frosch PJ, Kligman AM: The soap chamber test. J Am Acad Dermatol 1979;1:35.
20 Patrick E, Maibach HI: Dermatotoxicology; in Hayes AW (ed): Principles and Methods of Toxicology, ed 2. New York, Raven Press, 1989, pp 383–406.
21 Wilhelm KP, Wolff HH, Maibach HI: Effect of surfactants on skin hydration; in Elsner P, Berardesca E, Maibach HI (eds): Handbooks of Skin Bioengineering: Water and the Stratum corneum. Boca Raton. CRC Press 1994, vol 1, pp 257–274.

Klaus.-P. Wilhelm, MD, *proDERM* Institute for Applied Dermatological Research,
Industriestrasse 1, D–22869 Schenefeld/Hamburg (Germany)

Elsner P, Lachapelle JM, Wahlberg JE, Maibach HI (eds): Prevention of Contact Dermatitis. Curr Probl Dermatol. Basel, Karger, 1996, vol 25, pp 86–96

Allergy Caused by Acrylics: Past, Present and Prevention

L. Kanerva, T. Estlander, R. Jolanki

Finnish Institute of Occupational Health, Helsinki, Finland

The methacrylate and acrylate compounds, here called acrylics, were developed during the 1930s. They soon found extensive application in plastic glass (Plexiglas, Perspex, Lucite) for aircraft, interior and exterior house paints, coating for wood and paper, textile sizing, the treatment and finishing of textiles, printing, and floor polishes [1], as well as in dentistry [2–5].

1940s–1950s

In 1941, Stevenson [2] and Moody [3] were the first to report hypersensitivity from methyl methacrylate (MMA). In 1948, Bradford [4] had a patient with stomatitis from a dental methacrylate prosthesis. The patient showed an allergic patch test reaction with the prosthesis. In 1954, Fisher [5] encountered two dentists with dermatitis of the right hand, mainly of the first fingers, and two dental technicians with dermatitis of both hands. The dermatitis corresponded to what is seen today in dental and other personnel allergic to acrylics, i.e. fingertip dermatitis (fig. 1a). The patients of Fisher [5] had occupationally been sensitized to methacrylates, and had positive patch test reactions to undiluted MMA. Another currently common cause of allergic contact dermatitis (ACD) caused by acrylics, i.e. artificial nails [6, 7], was also reported already in the 1950s [8, 9].

Prevention. Schwartz et al. [10] advised in 1957 that 'the prevention of dermatitis among dental technicians from the resins used for making dentures consists of wearing rubber gloves and impervious sleeves and aprons', i.e. the preventive measures more or less used today, except that we now know that acrylics readily penetrate rubber gloves [11].

1960s–1970s

Allardize [12] was the first to report sensitization from acrylics in anaerobic sealers. By 1987, at least 119 cases had been reported [13].

The first case of allergy to bone cement made of acrylics was reported in an orthopedic surgeon by Pegum and Medhurst [11] in 1971. Fisher [14] reported five further orthopedic surgeons with occupational dermatitis in 1973, and all of them also complained of a burning type of paresthesia – a symptom common today in dental personnel [15, 16].

During the 1970s, there were outbreaks of dermatitis caused by UV-cured chemicals (partly acrylics) in the graphic industry from printing plates and inks [17]. These plastic photographic printing processes revolutionized the industry, but as only little was known about the sensitizing capacity of the chemicals used in UV printing, workers were not warned about the risks. At the Finnish Institute of Occupational Health (FIOH), printing plates and photo resins of Letterflex® (W.R. Grace and Company), Asahi photo resin (APR®, Asahi), Nyloprint® (BASF) and Ultracure® (Lorilleux) caused a total of 11 cases of ACD [18].

Prevention. Pegum and Medhurst [11] observed that MMA readily penetrates rubber gloves – a significant problem in the prevention of ACD caused by acrylics still today. At FIOH there were great difficulties in diagnosing and preventing occupational dermatoses, as the manufacturers were unwilling to reveal the chemicals used in, for example, the printing plates, and material safety data sheets (MSDS) were not mandatory. The Finnish Identification and Labelling System for Hazardous Chemicals (286/78) in 1978 has made MSDS mandatory, and contributed to the prevention of occupational dermatoses in Finland [18].

1980s

At FIOH, dental personnel have been found to have the highest number of occupational ACD from acrylics, probably because stronger sensitizers were taken into wider use in dentistry (dental composite resins and dentin primers). Our material (1980 to date) consists of 30 cases diagnosed as having occupational ACD from acrylics. All patients were patch tested with a European standard series and a (meth)acrylate series (table 1), and all patients showed an allergic patch test reaction to at least one of the acrylics. Dental composite resins, 12 cases, and dentin primers, 11 cases, were the most common causes of sensitization. Work with dental prostheses sensitized 6 persons, and work with hybrid glass-ionomers 1. The typical sign of initial

Table 1. Results of patch testing 124 patients with the (meth)acrylate series. From Kanerva et al. [21], with permission

	(Meth)acrylate series		% (w/w)	
1	Ethyl acrylate	(EA)	0.1–0.5	9/124 NG
2	Butyl acrylate	(BA)	0.1–0.5	6/124 NG
3	2-Ethylhexyl acrylate	(2-EHA)	0.1–0.5	0/124 V
4	2-Hydroxyethyl acrylate	(2-HEA)	0.1–0.5	14/124 NG
5	2-Hydroxypropyl acrylate	(2-HPA)	0.1–0.5	12/124 NG
6	Methyl methacrylate	(MMA)	2	8/124 NG
7	Ethyl methacrylate	(EMA)	2	6/124 NG
8	n-Butyl methacrylate	(BMA)	2	2/124 NG
9	2-Hydroxyethyl methacrylate	(2-HEMA)	2	13/124 I
10	2-Hydroxypropyl methacrylate	(2-HPMA)	2	15/124 I
11	Ethylene glycol dimethacrylate	(EGDMA)	2	11/124 I
12	Triethylene glycol dimethacrylate	(TREGDMA)	2	11/124 I
13	1,4-Butanediol dimethacrylate	(BUDMA)	2	4/124 I
14	Urethane dimethacrylate	(UEDMA)	2	0/124 II
15	2,2-bis[4-(2-Methacryloxyethoxy) phenyl]propane	(BIS-EMA)	1	2/124 IV
16	2,2-bis[4-(Methacryloxy)phenyl]propane	(BIS-MA)	2	0/124 V
17	2,2-bis[4-(2-Hydroxy-3-methacryloxypropoxy) phenyl]propane	(BIS-GMA)	2	4/124 I
18	1,4-Butanediol diacrylate	(BUDA)	0.1	6/124 III–V
19	1,6-Hexanediol diacrylate	(HDDA)	0.1	5/124 III–V
20	Diethylene glycol diacrylate	(DEGDA)	0.1	6/124 II
21	Tripropylene glycol diacrylate	(TPGDA)	0.1	0/124 IV
22	Trimethylolpropane triacrylate	(TMPTA)	0.1	0/124 IV
23	Pentaerythritol triacrylate	(PETA)	0.1	2/124 V
24	Oligotriacrylate 480	(OTA 480)	0.1	0/124 III
25	Epoxy diacrylate	(BIS-GA)	0.5	4/124 III–V
26	Urethane diacrylate (aliphatic)	(al-UDA)	0.1	0/124 V
27	Urethane diacrylate (aromatic)	(ar-UDA)	0.05	2/124 II
28	Triethylene glycol diacrylate	(TREGDA)	0.1	12/124 I
29	N,N-Methylene bis-acrylamide	(MBAA)	1	0/83 NG
30	Tetrahydrofurfuryl methacrylate	(THFMA)	2	2/16 NG

NG = Not given; I = weak; II = mild; III = moderate; IV = strong; V = extreme.

Twenty-three patients showed at least one allergic patch test reaction. The results have been compared to the sensitizing capacity of (meth)acrylates based on data obtained from animal studies according to Björkner [30].

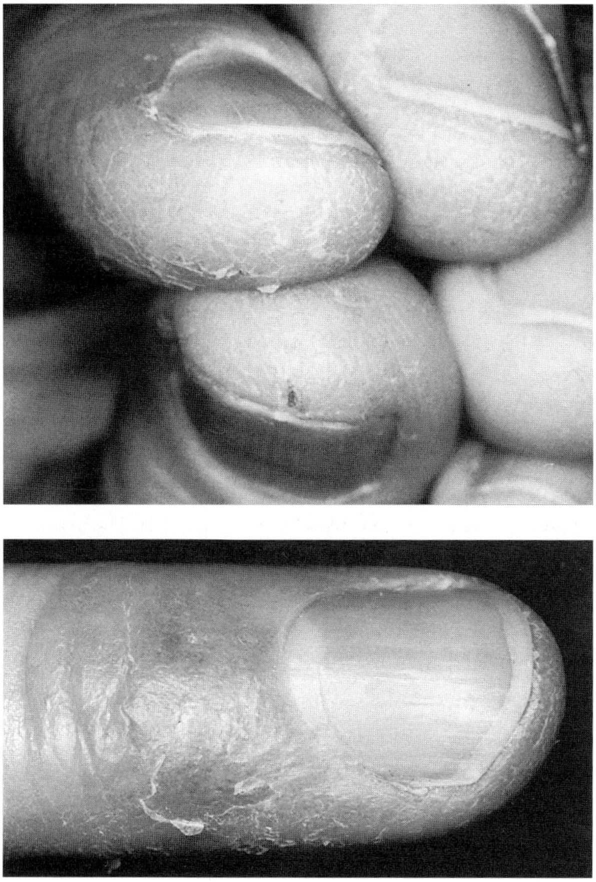

a

b

Fig. 1. *a* Typical initial fingertip dermatitis of a dentist allergic to acrylics. *b* Continued exposure results in extension of the dermatitis to the sides and back of the fingers. Same dentist as in (*a*).

allergic dermatitis was fingertip dermatitis (pulpitis; fig. 1a) but as exposure continued, the sides and the backs of the fingers also became involved (fig. 1b). Relapses were frequent and several patients were obliged to change jobs. More than half of the patients also developed paresthesia of the fingertips. Common acrylic sensitizers were 2-HEMA (the full names of the acrylics are given in table 1), dimethacrylates such as TREGDMA, and epoxy dimethacrylates such as BIS-GMA. MMA did not screen for allergy to acrylics as well as 2-HEMA. Gas chromatography/mass spectrometry (GC/MS) analysis showed that many undeclared acrylics are present in dental products, indicat-

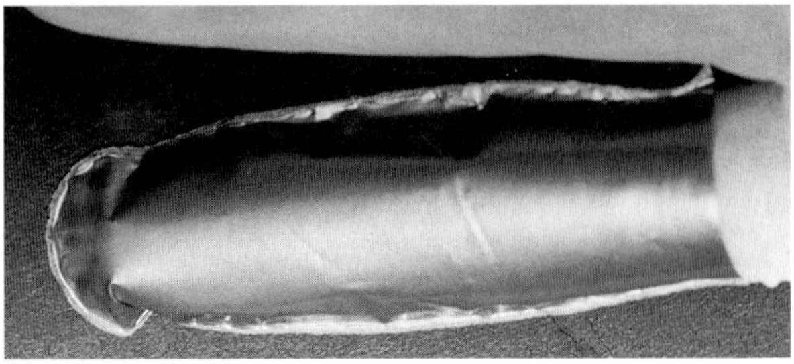

Fig. 2. Fingertip piece of laminated 4H glove can be used under or over a disposable latex or PVC glove to inhibit penetration of acrylics.

ing that MSDSs are not sufficiently accurate [16] (see below). Dental patients have on some occasions developed symptoms from dental composite resins or primers, and sensitized patients may be able to have dental fillings made of acrylics [19].

Prevention. A new glove material, 4-H-glove (fig. 2), a laminate composed of five layers, with a thickness of 0.065 mm has been introduced and shown to inhibit the penetration of, e.g., MMA and epoxy resins of the bisphenol-A-type [20].

1990s

Statistics

One hundred and twenty-four patients with a history of exposure to acrylate compounds were patch tested with conventional patch test techniques. Twenty-three showed at least one positive patch test reaction [21]. The three most often positive acrylate compounds were 2-HPMA, 2-HEA and 2-HEMA. The acrylate compounds that caused the most sensitizations are probably significant contact sensitizers in humans, or have a strong tendency to cross-react with sensitizers. There is not a good correlation between the sensitizing capacity of acrylics based on animal studies and our patch test results (table 1). The statistics in an American material were different, probably because of the different exposure history of the patients [6].

Aerobic Acrylic Adhesive

Anaerobic acrylic sealants containing polyethylene glycol dimethacrylates, are well-known sensitizers, but acrylate glues that cure in air have only seldom been reported as allergens. A patient sensitized to such a glue, and developing hand dermatitis that spread to the lower arms, chest, neck and face was examined at FIOH [22]. The glue was analyzed by GC/MS and found to contain 24.6% 2-HEMA and 0.4% EGDMA. These two acrylate compounds, as well as the glue, provoked an allergic patch test reaction. Also, many other acrylate compounds, e.g. THFMA, gave an allergic reaction indicating cross-allergy. The patient could not continue in her previous workplace because of severely relapsing skin symptoms.

Phenoxyethoxy Ethylacrylates

In an optical-fiber manufacturing plant the fibers were coated with UV-curable acrylic resin. After 2 months' work, a subject developed dermatitis. On patch testing the acrylate-coated fibers and the UV-curable acrylate coating resin provoked an allergic patch test reaction. Nineteen components of the acrylate coating were tested separately, and one component, namely phenoxy ethylacrylate, provoked allergic reactions at 0.1–0.0001% pet. Chemical analysis revealed it to contain 84% 2-phenoxy ethylacrylate and 12 other phenoxy-ethoxy ethylacrylates [23]. The same new allergens have recently been revealed in glues [23, 24].

Photobonded Sculptured Nails

A cosmetologist became occupationally sensitized from photobonded sculptured nails [7]. Table 2 shows some of the data that are needed for the complete diagnostics of allergy caused by acrylics: MSDS, CAS number, GC/MS and patch test results. The nail gel used for the photobonded nails contained 0.3% methyl acrylate (MA), 2% hydroxyethyl acrylate, 0.3% tripropylene glycol acrylate (TPGA) and 8% TPGDA (table 2). In the (meth)acrylate series 15 of the 31 (meth)acrylate compounds tested gave an allergic reaction: 2 acrylates, 5 methacrylates, 5 diacrylates and 3 dimethacrylates. Epoxy diacrylates, ethyl cyanoacrylate, triacrylates and methacrylic acid were negative. Three of seven of her own nail cosmetic preparations contained mono(meth)acrylates as revealed by the GC/MS, and these also gave allergic patch test reactions, namely the nail liquid, nail hardener, and the UV-cured nail gel (table 2). The patient had probably been sensitized to the following acrylics from her nail cosmetics: TPGDA and MA from her photobonded nail gel; EMA, TREGDMA and MMA from her nail liquid, and BMA from her nail hardener. She was probably also sensitized to the rare sensitizer al-UDA (table 1). As nail cosmetics containing acrylics are strong sensitizers, both the workers and the customers should be aware of their sensitizing capacity; they should use no-touch techniques as regards the skin, before the mono(meth)acrylates are polymerized.

Table 2. Patch test results and composition of a patient's own substances according to gas chromatography/mass spectrometry analysis, and material safety data sheets (MSDS): from Kanerva et al. [7], with permission

Product	Use	MSDS or product declaration sheet		CAS number	GC/MS analysis	%	Patch test result (concentration, in pet)
Professionals powder	polymer powder for sculptured nails	poly ethyl methacrylate ethyl methacrylate homopolymer		9003–42–3	methyl methacrylate ethyl methacrylate	0.2 0.6	neg. (as is)
Professionals liquid	monomer liquid for sculptured nails	ethyl methacrylate MEHQ benzophenone	>98 0.002 <2	97–63–2 150–76–5 131–57–7	methyl methacrylate ethyl methacrylate triethylene glycol dimethacrylate	0.5 90 5	2+ 2% 2+ 0.64% 1+ 0.2%
Develop 10 program for strong nails	nail strengthener	butyl acetate; ethyl acetate; toluol; nitrocellulose; isopropanol; dibutyl phthalate; toluene sulfonamide methanal polymer (formaldehyde resin); hydrolyzed protein; DMDM hydantoin; FD&C violet No. 2		n.a.	N-butylmethacrylate methyl acrylate	2.2 <0.5	2+ (as is; hardened) neg. 5%
Develop 10 beautiful colors	nail lacquer	butyl acetate; toluene; nitrocellulose; ethyl acetate; toluenesulfonamide methanal polymer (formaldehyde resin); dibutyl phthalate; isopropanol; steralkonium hectorate; camphor; benzophenone-1; DMDM hydantoin; polyester resin		n.a.	methyl acrylate	<0.5	2+ (as is; hardened) 1+ 10
Nail primer	primer	methacrylic acid other ester addvets MEHQ	<98.5 <1.5 trace	n.a.	methacrylic acid methyl methacrylate	88 0.1	neg. 1% neg. 0.32% neg. 0.1%
APC UV nail gel	UV-cured nail gel	acrylate ester of bisphenol a based epoxy tripropylene glycol diacrylate	 <10	H 055818–57–0* H 042978–60–5	methyl acrylate hydroxyethyl acrylate tripropylene glycol acrylate tripropylene glycol diacrylate	0.3 2 0.3 8	2+ 1% 2+ 0.32% 2+ 0.1%
Glue	for tips and wraps	cyanoacrylate		n.a.	acrylates	<0.05%	neg. 1%

n.a. = Not available; neg. = negative; MEHQ = mono methyl ether hydroquinone = 4-methoxyphenol; DMDM hydantoin = dimetylol dimethyl hydantoin; benzophenone = benzophenone 3 = 2-hydroxy-4-methoxybenzophenone; * = BIS-GMA.

Table 3. Major factors in the prevention of occupational dermatoses

1	Identification of potential irritants and allergens
2	Engineering controls
3	Chemical substitution
4	Personal protection: protective gloves, clothing, barrier creams
5	Good personal and environmental hygiene
6	Regulation of allergens and irritants within the workplace
7	Education; awareness of allergens and irritants
8	Motivational techniques to establish safe work conditions
9	Pre-employment and periodic health screening
10	Accurate material safety data sheets
11	Updated instructions for use
12	Chemical and personal protective measures
13	Legislative regulations, directives

Tri-Cure Glass Ionomer

A dental hygienist developed finger dermatitis. Patch testing indicated that the sources were a dentin primer and a new tri-cure glass ionomer [25]. The latter has not been reported earlier to cause allergy to acrylics. The sensitizer in the glass ionomer was 2-HEMA, currently one of the most common sensitizers in dental products [25].

Occupational Asthma

Acrylic resins may cause asthma. Eighteen cases have been reported from our Institute [26]. Cyanoacylates have been the most common cause, but also methacrylates have provoked asthma. Prick testing has been negative in all cases, and the mechanisms of the hypersensitivity reactions are not known. The diagnosis is based on chamber provocation tests.

It should be emphasized that the first case report of OACD from dental composite acrylic resins was not published until 1993 in the USA [27], indicating significant underreporting and underdiagnostics of this epidemic in the USA.

Prevention. Good advice to prevent occupational contact dermatitis is available in the literature [28], (table 3). Regarding acrylics, many problems have not yet been solved satisfactorily. We have suggested that dental products containing acrylics should be delivered in such bottles/packagings that the no-touch techniques could be used while handling acrylics [29], but currently this is not the case [25]. Identification of acrylic allergens can be performed with GC/MS analysis [16], and accurate MSDSs/product declarations should

Table 4. Material safety data sheets may be inaccurate because of the following factors

1	Low concentrations of chemicals are not declared
2	Raw materials may contain hidden impurities
3	Final product may contain starting materials
4	Decomposition of components
5	Contamination or residues from packaging
6	Manufacturing process may be poorly controlled
7	Undeclared components may be added intentionally

be required from the industry before the products are sold; otherwise many patients/customers will be sensitized before any preventive measures have taken place.

Good advice on acrylic substitution may currently be difficult to give, because animal studies and human experiences are not in good agreement. For example, one of the most common sensitizers in humans, 2-HEMA, is a weak sensitizer in animals according to Björkner [30] (table 1).

Rubber gloves are readily penetrated by acrylics [11], and the 4-H glove is not of good anatomic fit for delicate tasks. We have therefore suggested that a fingerpiece of the 4H glove under a disposable glove may be used, for example, by dental personnel. Another possibility is to use the fingerpiece on the disposable glove (fig. 2), as suggested by one of our sensitized dentists. MSDSs were not available in Finland before 1978, and this caused great problems when trying to identify the sensitizers in more sophisticated industries because of the unwillingness of the manufacturers to cooperate. MSDSs today are of great help, but from an allergist's point of view they may not be exact (table 4). We feel that a great effort should be directed towards more complete MSDSs, and the allergist also needs to know the components with a lower concentration than 1%. Currently, chemicals with a concentration below 1% are not usually declared even when they are allergenic.

References

1 Adams RM: Occupational Contact Dermatitis. Philadelphia, Lippincott, 1969.

2 Stevenson WJ: Methyl-methacrylate dermatitis. Contact Point 1941;18:171–173.

3 Moody WL: Severe reaction from acrylic liquid. Dent Digest 1941;47:305.

4 Bradford EW: Case of allergy to methyl-methacrylate. Br Dent J 1948;84:195.

5 Fisher AA: Allergic sensitisation of the skin and oral mucosa to acrylic denture materials. JAMA 1954;156:238–242.

6 Koppula SV, Fellman JH, Storrs FJ: Screening for acrylate dermatitis associated with artificial nails. Am J Contact Dermatitis 1995;6:78–85.

7 Kanerva L, Lauerma A, Estlander T, Alanko K, Jolanki R: Occupational allergic contact dermatitis caused by photobonded sculptured nails and a review on (meth)acrylates in nail cosmetics. Am J Contact Dermatitis 1996;in press.

8 Canizares O: Contact dermatitis due to the acrylic materials used in artificial nails. Arch Dermatol 1956;74:141–143.

9 Fisher AA, Franks A, Glick H: Allergic sensitization of the skin and nails to acrylic plastic nails. J Allergy 1957;28:84.

10 Schwartz L, Tulipan L, Peck SM: Occupational Diseases of the Skin, ed 2. London, Henry Kimpton, 1957, p 476.

11 Pegum JS, Medhurst FA: Contact dermatitis from penetration of rubber gloves by acrylic monomer. Br Med J 1971;ii:141.

12 Allardize JT: Dermatitis due to an acrylic resin sealer. Trans St Johns Hosp Dermatol Soc 1967; 53:86–89.

13 Kanerva L, Estlander T, Jolanki R: Occupational allergic contact dermatitis from acrylates: Observations concerning anaerobic sealants and dental composite resins, in Frosch PJ, et al (eds): Current Topics in Contact Dermatitis. Berlin, Springer, 1989, pp 352–359.

14 Fisher AA: Acrylic bone cement sensitization and dermatitis. Cutis 1973;12:333–337.

15 Kanerva L, Estlander T, Jolanki R: Allergic contact dermatitis from dental composite resins due to aromatic epoxy acrylates and aliphatic acrylates. Contact Dermatitis 1989;20:201–211.

16 Kanerva L, Henriks-Eckerman M-L, Estlander T, Jolanki R, Tarvainen K: Occupational allergic contact dermatitis and composition of acrylates in dentin bonding systems. J Eur Acad Derm Venereol 1994;3:157–268.

17 Malten KE, Bende WJM: 2-Hydroxy-ethyl-methacrylate and di- and tetraethylene glycol dimethacrylate: Contact sensitizers in a photopolymer printing plate procedure. Contact Dermatitis 1979;5:214.

18 Kanerva L, Estlander T, Jolanki R, Sysilampi M-L: Allergy caused by acrylate compounds: History, research and prevention. People Work Res Rep 1995;4:135–138.

19 Kanerva L, Alanko K: Stomatitis and perioral dermatitis caused by epoxy diacrylates in dental composite resins. J Am Acad Derm, in press.

20 Roed-Petersen J: A new glove material protective against epoxy and acrylate monomer; in Frosch PJ, et al (eds): Current Topics in Contact Dermatitis. Berlin, Springer, 1989, pp 603–606.

21 Kanerva L, Estlander T, Jolanki K: Statistics on allergic patch test reactions caused by acrylate compounds, including data on ethyl methacrylate. Am J Contact Dermatitis 1995;6:1–4.

22 Kanerva L, Jolanki R, Leino T, Estlander T: Occupational allergic contact dermatitis from 2-hydroxyethyl methacrylate and ethylene glycol dimethacrylate in a modified acrylic structural adhesive. Contact Dermatitis 1995;33:84–89.

23 Jolanki R, Estlander T, Suhonen R, Henriks-Eckerman M-L, Kanerva L: Contact allergy to phenoxyethoxy ethylacrylates. 2nd Congr Euro Soc Contact Dermatitis, Barcelona, 6–8 October, 1994, p 60.

24 Busschots AM, Meuleman V, Poesen N, Dooms-Goossens A: Contact allergy to components of glue in insulin infusion sets. Contact Dermatitis 1995;33:205–206.

25 Kanerva L, Estlander T, Jolanki R, Koskinen KP: Lasi-ionomeerin ja 2-hydroksimetakrylaatin (2-HEMAn) aiheuttama allerginen työperäinen käsi-ihottuma erikoishammashoitajalla. (Occupational allergic contact dermatitis in a dental nurse caused by light cured hybrid glass ionomer and 2-hydroxyethylmethacrylate (2-HEMA).) Suomen Hammaslääkl 1995;5:234–236. (Finnish Dental Journal, in Finnish with English abstract, p 284.)

26 Savonius B, Keskinen H, Tuppurainen M, Kanerva L: Occupational respiratory disease caused by acrylates. Clin Exp Allergy 1993;23:416–424.

27 Johnson DR, Mathias CGT: Case report: A dentist with allergic contact dermatitis caused by ethylene glycol dimethacrylate. Am J Contact Dermatitis 1993;4:90–92.

28 Lachapelle J-M: Principles of prevention and protection in contact dermatitis (with special reference to occupational dermatology); in Rycroft RJG, et al (eds): Textbook of Contact Dermatitis, ed 2. Berlin, Springer, 1995, pp 695–702.

29 Kanerva L, Turjanmaa K, Estlander T, Jolanki R: Occupational allergic contact dermatitis from 2-hydroxyethyl methacrylate (2-HEMA) in a new dentin adhesive. Am J Contact Dermatitis 1991; 2:24–30.

30 Björkner B: Kontaktallergi för ultraviolett härdande akrylatprodukter i färger och lacker. Arbete och Hälsa 1989;20:1–39.

Prof. Lasse Kanerva, Section of Dermatology, Finnish Institute of Occupational Health, Topeliuksenkatu 41 aA, FIN–00250 Helsinki (Finland)

Elsner P, Lachapelle JM, Wahlberg JE, Maibach HI (eds): Prevention of Contact Dermatitis. Curr Probl Dermatol. Basel, Karger, 1996, vol 25, pp 97–105

Prevention by Exposure Assessment

Mari-Ann Flyvholm

Department of Occupational Medicine, National Institute of Occupational Health, Copenhagen, Denmark

Exposure assessment is important in the prevention of allergic contact dermatitis. This chapter focuses on exposure to contact allergens from chemical products and will briefly go through the need for information and some investigations showing the value of exposure information and then it will focus on the sources of information on exposure. Knowledge of exposure is important for all procedures related to the management of allergic contact dermatitis from the clinical investigation and treatment and the following guidance of the sensitized eczema patients to the prevention of new cases of sensitization in the healthy part of the general population.

The need for exposure assessment or exposure information is frequently emphasized in the literature [1–3]. In a section on 'Principles of prevention and protection in contact dermatitis' in the 'Textbook of Contact Dermatitis' Lachapelle [1] says that: 'A better knowledge of the chemical nature of the various products used at work is of prime importance. Needless to say, such information is difficult to acquire in many instances. . . .'

Another example is from Veien's [2] thesis on eczema. Instead of positive patch test results which were listed as being of unknown relevance, '. . .more patients might have received a final diagnosis of allergic contact dermatitis had we known more about the presence in the environment of the substances in question'. This is critical as the further management of eczema differs for patients with irritant contact dermatitis and patients with allergic contact dermatitis. Sensitized patients with allergic contact dermatitis depend on the ability to eliminate or reduce further contact with the offending allergen.

Furthermore, several studies have shown that patients with allergic contact dermatitis can benefit from exposure assessment which is used for careful instruction concerning the occurrence of contact allergens in products for industrial, household or personal use [4–7].

Cronin [4] investigated formaldehyde sensitized eczema patients. For a group of patients with 'domestic exposure' the exposure to formaldehyde from cleaning agents was investigated based on product lists and inquiries to suppliers. Formaldehyde exposure was found in 20 of 21 patients and the patients were advised to use formaldehyde-free products. 'The improvement in their hand eczema was unexpectedly good.'

In a study on formaldehyde-sensitized eczema patients the assessment of exposure to chemical products (occupational, household, personal care and cosmetics) was made as a supplement to the normal dermatological consultation. This investigation included an interview with a chemist, listing of all products used by the patients, and product screening by use of a product data base. The study showed that all patients were exposed to products containing formaldehyde or formaldehyde releasers. After elimination of exposure this secondary prevention was successful for 2/3 of the patients as their eczema healed or improved to a degree making further consultations unnecessary [5].

In a study on the causes of occupational skin diseases in Finland an increasing number of patients were diagnosed as allergic eczema after having included an interview with a chemist and it was noted that 'consultations with a chemist have proved to be of great importance in revealing suspected allergens' [6].

Thus, there is an unsatisfied need for information on the occurrence of contact allergens and as mentioned above investigations have shown that information on exposure can improve the prognosis for eczema patients.

Primary and Secondary Prevention

Prevention of allergic contact dermatitis can be divided into primary and secondary prevention: primary prevention focuses on induction of contact sensitization and controlling the exposure which eventually lead to sensitization, and secondary prevention focuses on elicitation of allergic contact dermatitis (table 1). The measures for primary and secondary prevention can differ in some respects, but in several instances exposure assessment made for secondary prevention provides the knowledge necessary for initiation of measures for primary prevention, and the measures for primary prevention may constitute the secondary prevention by preventing new outbreaks of eczema in sensitized individuals.

Primary prevention can be to remove a contact allergen by use of alternative products, by changing the product composition or by changing the manu-

Table 1. Measures for primary and secondary prevention of allergic contact dermatitis

Primary prevention: prevent induction of contact sensitization	
Remove contact allergens	use alternative products change the product composition change the manufacturing process
Reduce or control the exposure	legal regulation change the use of the products
Secondary prevention: prevent elicitation of contact sensitization	
Diagnostic procedures	patch test series information on the relevance of positive patch test reactions
Information systems	product labelling leaflets on product types or occupations data bases

facturing process. For the consumer the change of products will normally mean a change to other products not containing the allergen in question. Manufacturers can act by changing the product composition or by changing the manufacturing process causing the content of allergenic substances. Another type of primary prevention is to reduce or control the exposure by legislation concerning the concentration of contact allergens in products or by changing the use of products.

In the secondary prevention exposure information is needed in the diagnostic procedures in order to formulate patch test series, or as information to decide which allergens to test with or to reveal the relevance of positive patch test reactions. Information systems (labelling, leaflets and data bases) can provide information to patients and doctors in order to identify where exposure to the specific allergen occur both in the home and in the occupational environment.

Exposure Assessment

In general, measures of prevention of allergic contact dermatitis require exposure assessment at some stage in the procedure and exposure assessment requires methods to supply information on exposure. The following is an overview on different methods or sources of information available for exposure assessment.

Table 2. Sources of information on exposure to chemical contact allergens – limitations and advantages

Product labelling	direct accessible limited by information available, source of allergen etc.
Chemical analysis	effective if methods are available can be simple and quick problematic for complex products
Inquiries to manufacturers or suppliers	can cost extensive resources and time delay lack of specific information
Product data bases	can be simple and quick can provide information on specific products or cross-sectional for a substance detailed information and updating can be a problem access may be limited

Sources of information on exposure can be divided into: product labelling, chemical analysis, inquiries to manufacturers or suppliers and product data bases. Each have their limitations and advantages depending on the type of product, the suspected allergen, and the source of the allergen (table 2). The information may be (old) 'textbook knowledge' or based on the latest scientific papers but even in such cases sources of information have been required at some stage.

Product Labelling

Product labelling is essential for both primary and secondary prevention [8] and this is the only type of information which is directly available provided a minimum of ability to read and interpret chemical names is at hand.

Labelling is limited to the information available, to the manufacturers making the labelling and by the legal demands to the labelling. In the USA, cosmetics have been labelled with lists of components for several years [9, 10]. A new EC Cosmetic Directive will require labelling of cosmetics with lists of ingredients except for perfumes [11]. The value of the European product labelling is limited as components occurring in products in concentrations below 1% (which is 10,000 ppm) are not declared. Components added to raw materials or ingredients used in the manufacturing process may be missing in the labelling. Labelling requirements have to include all ingredients and all types of products for personal, domestic and occupational use, etc.

Chemical Analysis

In the detection of well-defined and known substances chemical analysis is an effective way to obtain information on the occurrence of contact allergens provided that reliable analytical methods exist for the allergen in question. The ideal situation is that simple and quick test methods can be performed in the laboratories of the dermatological departments. If the methods are complicated or require equipment which is not available in an ordinary laboratory of a dermatological department the use of commercial laboratories may add unrealistic costs and time delay to the procedure. To give a few examples, nickel in metal objects can be detected by the dimethylglyoxime test and formaldehyde can be detected by the chromotropic acid test and the acetylacetone test [12, 13].

Without a precise knowledge of which substances to look out for chemical analysis is problematic to use as it can be difficult in complex products. Further development and validation of simple analytical methods is needed.

Inquiries to Manufacturers or Suppliers

The use of inquiries to manufacturers or suppliers as a tool in exposure assessment can be very difficult and the time delay is often a major problem. Sometimes specific chemical information is not available from the manufacturers. When this is the case, inquiries to manufacturers are not a usable method in the daily routine due to the use of resources and the time delay. Some manufacturers, however, are cooperative and able to supply detailed information quickly and may even provide information on the specific batch used.

Product Data Bases

Product data bases with computerized information on chemical products can be a quick and simple way to obtain information on the composition of specific products causing eczema or cross-sectional information on the occurrence of specific allergenic substances [14, 15]. Product data bases can be used as information systems which provide knowledge on the occurrence of contact allergens to both patients and doctors – or as a tool to survey the use of chemicals and planning the preventive measures. Although, the product categories included in the data bases, the degree of details and the updating of the registration often causes limitations in the usefulness. This, in combination with restrictions in access if the registered information is confidential, may be the reason why the data bases are not used in an 'optimal' way by dermatologists and other doctors.

National product data bases based on legal demands to manufacturers or importers for notifying hazardous products exist in Denmark (PROBAS)

Table 3. Sources of formaldehyde in products

Components
Hidden content from raw materials
Residues from synthesis
Decomposition of components
Packages coated with formaldehyde resins

[16, 17], Sweden [18] and Norway [19]. In the USA nationwide surveys provide data bases with information on the composition of occupational products (NOHS: National Occupational Hazard Survey and NOES: National Occupational Exposure Survey) [20–24]. A national survey on the use of chemicals [25] has been included in the Danish national data base – The Danish Product Register (PROBAS). Data bases with information on specific product categories are available in, for example, the USA for cosmetics (FDA) [26–28] and for occupational products (EPA) [29, 30]. Data bases run by dermatological departments exist, for example, in Belgium (Codex) [31], Finland (INFODERM) [32], Sweden (DALUK) [33] and Italy (OCCALL) [34].

With formaldehyde used as an example, it can be seen that different causes of formaldehyde in products require different sources of information (table 3). Normally product labelling with information on components will only provide information on components added on purpose. Chemical analysis will include occurrence of the substances irrespective of their origin. Inquiries to manufacturers or suppliers will often be restricted to the components added and sometimes raw materials, residues, decomposition and contamination from packages (if analyzed). Product data bases will provide knowledge on components and raw materials and maybe residues and decomposition. Thus, among other things the value of the different sources of information depends on the source of the allergen in question.

Conclusion

The exposure assessment provides a part of the knowledge needed for prevention. We are operating somewhere in the field of or chain from basic knowledge on health hazards to the outcome we want – which is fewer skin diseases – and a lot of things have to be changed before we see the results. The preventive measures to control or reduce exposure to contact allergens depend on the occurrence of the chemical in focus. The ways of preventing

Table 4. Ways of preventing contact sensitization

1	Replace
	Certain chemicals
	Particular products
2	Regulate exposure to sensitizing chemicals
	Generally
	In specific products
	In particular work processes or businesses
3	Provide optimal information
	Diagnostic systems
	Information systems
	Education of groups or individuals
4	Individually oriented preventive methods
	Gloves
	Barrier creams
	Protective clothing

Adapted from Menné et al. [35].

contact sensitization, shown in table 4, were drawn up in a paper on 'Prevention of allergic contact sensitization to chemicals' [35]. Common environmental chemicals frequently used both in domestic and occupational products need to be legally regulated by replacement (substitution) or concentration limits. Chemicals used in specific work processes or businesses can be controlled by encapsulation, ventilation, education of the workers or use of personal protective equipment.

References

1 Lachapelle J-M: Principles of prevention and protection in contact dermatitis; in Rycroft RJG, Menné T, Frosch PJ, Benezra C (eds): Textbook of Contact Dermatitis. Berlin, Springer, 1992, pp 695–702.

2 Veien NK: Systemically induced eczema in adults. Acta Derm Venereol Suppl (Stockh) 1989;147: 1–58.

3 Wahlberg JE: Patch testing; in Rycroft RJG, Menné T, Frosch PJ, Benezra C (eds): Textbook of Contact Dermatitis. Berlin, Springer, 1992, pp 241–268.

4 Cronin E: Formaldehyde is a significant allergen in women with hand eczema. Contact Dermatitis 1991;25:276–282.

5 Flyvholm M-A, Menné T: Allergic contact dermatitis from formaldehyde: A case study focussing on sources of formaldehyde exposure. Contact Dermatitis 1992;27:27–36.

6 Estlander T: Occupational skin disease in Finland: Observations made during 1974–1988 at the Institute of Occupational Health, Helsinki, Acta Derm Venereol Suppl (Stockh) 1990;155: 1–85.

7 Edman B: The usefulness of detailed information to patients with contact allergy. Contact Dermatitis 1988;19:43–47.

8 Flyvholm M-A, Menné T, Maibach HI: Exposures and dose-response relationships; in: Vos JG, Younes M, Smith E (eds): Allergic Hypersensitivities Induced by Chemicals. Recommendations for Prevention. Boca Raton, CRC Press, 1995, pp 261–285.

9 Larsen WG: Why is the USA the only country with compulsory cosmetic labeling. Contact Dermatitis 1989;20:1–2.

10 De Groot AC, White IR: Cosmetic ingredient labelling in the European Community. Contact Dermatitis 1991;25:273–275.

11 Council Directive 93/35/EEC of 14 June 1993 amending for the sixth time Directive 76/768/EEC on the approximation of the laws of the Member States relating to cosmetic products. Official Journal No L 325, 23/06/93 P 0024.

12 Fregert S, Björkner B, Bruze M, Dahlquist I, Gruvberger B, Persson K, Trulsson L, Zimerson E: Yrkesdermatologi, Lund, Studentlitteratur, 1990.

13 Fregert S: Physicochemical methods for detection of contact allergens; in Menné T, Maibach HI (eds): Exogenous Dermatoses: Environmental Dermatitis. Boston, CRC Press, 1991, pp 74–83.

14 Flyvholm M-A: Contact allergens in registered chemical products. Contact Dermatitis 1991;25: 49–56.

15 Flyvholm M-A: Positive patch-test results of unknown relevance explained by a database on chemical products. Proc 9th Int Symp Contact Dermatitis, 17–19 May 1990, Stockholm, Sweden. Contact Dermatitis 1990;23:285.

16 Danish Ministry of Labour: Order No 466 of 14th September 1981 on the Register of Substances and Materials. Copenhagen, Danish Ministry of Labour, 1984.

17 Flyvholm M-A, Andersen P, Beck ID, Brandorff NP: PROBAS: The Danish Product Register Data Base – a national register of chemical substances and products. J Hazardous Materials 1992; 30:59–69.

18 Statens naturvårdsverk: Produktkontroll. Kundgörelse om produktanmälan. SNFS 1979: 2 PK, Sweden, Statens naturvårdsverks författningssamling, 1979.

19 Produktregistret: Deklarering av kjemiske stoffer og produkter. Veiledning, Oslo, Produktregistret, 1989.

20 Seta JA, Sundin DS, Pedersen DH: National occupational exposure survey. Field guidelines. DHHS (NIOSH) Publ No 88-016. Cincinnati, US Department of Health & Human Services, 1988.

21 Sundin DS, Pedersen DH, Frazier TM: Occupational hazard and health surveillance. Am J Publ Health 1986;76:1083–1084.

22 Sundin DS: The national occupational hazard survey: A difficult quest for a reliable data base. Occup Health Saf 1978;47:21–23.

23 Sundin DS, Frazier TM: VII. Hazard surveillance at NIOSH. Am J Publ Health 1989;79:32–37.

24 Sieber WK Jr, Sundin DS, Frazier TM, Robinson CF: Development, use, and availability of a job exposure matrix based on national occupational hazard survey data. Am J Industr Med 1991;20: 163–174.

25 Brandorff NP, Flyvholm M-A, Beck ID, Skov T, Bach E: National survey on the use of chemicals in the working environment: Estimated exposure events. Occup Environ Med 1995;52: 454–463.

26 Richardson EL: Update: Frequency of preservative use in cosmetic formulas as disclosed to FDA. Cosmet Toilet 1981;96:91–92.

27 Decker RL: Frequency of preservative use in cosmetics as disclosed to FDA – 1984. Cosmet Toilet 1985;100:65–68.

28 Decker RL, Wenninger JA: Frequency of preservative use in cosmetic formulas as disclosed to FDA – 1987. Cosmet Toilet 1987;102:21–24.

29 White R: DERM/IONFONET: The American Academy of Dermatology's computer based information system for the clinical dermatologist; in: Dermatology in Five Continents. Proc XVII World Congr Dermatology, Berlin, May 24–29, 1987. Berlin, Springer, 1987, pp 831–832.

30 Kopf AW, Rigel DS, White R, Rosenthal L, Jordan WP, Carter DM, Everet MA, Moore J: DERM/INFONET: A concept becomes a reality. J Am Acad Dermatol 1988;18:1150–1157.

31 Drieghe J, Dooms-Goossens A, Dooms M, Degreef H: The Codex system. Semin Dermatol 1989; 8:96.

32 Rantanen T: INFODERM: A microcomputer database system with Finnish product files. Semin Dermatol 1989;8:94–95.

33 Edman B: DALUK: The Swedish computer system for contact dermatitis. Semin Dermatol 1989; 8:97–98.

34 Nava C, Venturi A, Meregalli E, Bon E, Beretta E: Information system in assessment of occupational allergy: The model of the institute of occupational health of Milan; in Parmeggiani L, Roi R, Aresini G, Bino G (eds): Proc 1st Int Workshop on Data Banks in Occupational Health, Villa Ponti, Varese, Italy, October 30/31, 1986. Ispra, EUR Ed, 1987, pp 192–203.

35 Menné T, Flyvholm M-A, Maibach HI: Prevention of allergic contact sensitization to chemicals; in: Vos JG, Younes M, Smith E (eds): Allergic Hypersensitivities Induced by Chemicals. Recommendations for Preventions. Boca Raton, CRC Press, 1995, pp 287–297.

Mari-Ann Flyvholm, MSc, PhD, Senior scientist, Department of Occupational Medicine,
National Institute of Occupational Health, Lersø Parkallé 105,
DK–2100 Copenhagen (Denmark)

Elsner P, Lachapelle JM, Wahlberg JE, Maibach HI (eds): Prevention of Contact Dermatitis. Curr Probl Dermatol. Basel, Karger, 1996, vol 25, pp 106–115

Predictive Testing of Metalworking Fluids and Development of Contact Dermatitis in Metalworkers

W. Wigger-Alberti[a], *U. Hinnen*[a,b], *P. Elsner*[a]

[a] Department of Dermatology and
[b] Institute of Social and Preventive Medicine, University of Zurich, Switzerland

Metal working fluids (MWF) used for cooling and lubrication during the machining process are one of the most important causes of hand dermatitis in the metal industry. Although computerized tooling operations are increasing, machinists still have contact with MWF frequently during adjusting machine tools. Two types of MWF are used: neat oils, used as extreme-pressure additives or corrosion inhibitor and water-based fluids, mixtures of mineral oils, organic acids, amines, emulsifiers, preservatives, biocides, anti-foams, fragrances and system cleaners [1]. All of these components may be irritants. Water-based MWF have a higher irritating and sensitizing potential than neat oils which are more likely to cause oil acne than eczema [1–4]. In spite of the irritating potential of MWF, predictive skin risk testing is done only sporadically and in different manners by MWF suppliers [5].

Epidemiology

Dermatitis from MWFs is usually irritant or multifactorial [1, 6]. The perception that irritant contact dermatitis (ICD) is more frequent than allergic contact dermatitis (ACD) due to MWF exposure is supported by data from Holland. In an unselected population of 286 metalworkers exposed to MWF, the vast majority of hand dermatitis cases were of the irritant type (14%) [1]. An allergological examination showed a contact sensitization in 2.8% of these workers [7]. Even if some authors [4, 8, 9] stated that ACD could represent

50% of the total, it is necessary to bear in mind that MWFs could act first as irritants and allow penetration of potential sensitizer through damaged skin [10]. This is also true for micro trauma from metal chips. A retrospective study of the epidemiology of occupational skin disease among metalworkers in Singapore showed that ICD (75%) prevailed over ACD [11]. In a prospective study, the cumulative incidence of occupational dermatitis from MWF among metalworkers in a metal fabrication factory remained at about 50% after a 6-month period [12]. Diepgen et al. [13] studied the incidence of occupational skin diseases in Northern Bavaria. Metalworkers had a high incidence of occupational skin diseases that was only outpassed by hairdressers. The risk for hand dermatitis in metalworkers is closely linked to MWF exposure. The prevalence of hand dermatitis may reach 30% if high MWF exposure is given [14]. Hinnen and Elsner [15] showed that 10% of Swiss metal worker trainees suffered from minor signs of skin irritation (erythema, induration, flaking) 8–10 months after the beginning of the apprenticeship and transepidermal water loss (TEWL) values rose continuously within 3 months of the first examination. The observed increase was significantly influenced only by exposure to water-soluble MWF.

Predictive Testing of MWF

In order to evaluate the risk a substance has to cause contact dermatitis a number of tests like in vitro assays, guinea pig sensitization tests, mouse sensitization tests as well as human sensitization assays have been developed. The risk of ICD is examined by in vitro assays as well as skin irritation tests in animals and humans [16]. More specifically, in recent studies different models have been proposed to evaluate the irritant effect of MWF quantitatively by noninvasive measuring methods. In an animal model, Goh investigated the effect of barrier creams [17] and emollient creams [18] on cutting oil dermatitis on guinea pig skin. He showed that 2 tested barrier creams and 2 'after-work' emollient creams appeared to aggravate the irritant effect of MWF on guinea pig skin.

In a human model, de Boer et al. [19] showed that MWF are generally only mildly irritant in their test procedure. They performed a repeated patch test on the volar area of the forearms over 5 days and evaluated the irritation of MWF and their components by a visual score and by laser Doppler flowmetry (table 1). Hüner et al. [20] proposed a single 24-hour patch test and repeated patch test (72 h) on the volar side of the right forearm to evaluate 3 MWF from different manufacturers. They showed that in spite of their similar alkalinity 2 of 3 MWF caused a significant increase in TEWL after a 24-hour occlusive

Table 1. Predictive testing of MWF

Author	Substances	Application	Measurement	Irritant reaction
de Boer et al. [19]	3 water-based MWF 2 neat oils (NO)	forearm patch test 24 h/4 × 12 h	visual score skin blood flow	water-based MWF > NO only 1 MWF > water
Hüner et al. [20]	3 water-based MWF	forearm patch test 24 h/72 h	visual Score TEWL skin blood flow	2 of 3 MWF > water

application and after cumulative exposure (table 1). In a field study, Coenraads et al. [21] performed weekly TEWL measurements during a 12-week working period in exposed and unexposed metal industry workers. They found TEWL to be and adequate tool for monitoring metalworkers exposed to mineral oils and MWF but they did not compare different products in the field setting.

Comparative Evaluation of Testing Methods

So far, no standard procedures exist for predictive skin irritancy testing of MWFs. This may be the reason why some Swiss suppliers of MWF products do not perform any sensitization testing or any cumulative irritation testing before marketing new MWF, and if so only a part of the products are tested [5]. The methods of testing are very heterogeneous: animal testing, human testing or a combination of both.

The aim of our study was to determine the irritancy of 3 different MWF by means of 2 different types of predictive tests. Based on the irritancy rating of 3 MWF by a prospective epidemiological field study in metalworking trainees, we performed a comparative study of 2 predictive tests for MWF irritancy in order to identify a sensitive and specific test that could be recommended for future testing.

Patients and Methods

Field Study

In the ongoing Prospective Metal Workers' Eczema Study (PROMETES) performed in cooperation between the Departments of Dermatology and Social and Preventive Medicine, University of Zurich, 205 metalworker trainees were nonselectively recruited in the trainees workshops of 22 different metalworking factories. They underwent an initial skin examination, including a standardised interview and a clinical examination of the skin. Dermal exposure assessment was based on expert interviews and job diaries. The trainees were reexamined 8–10 months after they had started their apprenticeship and all signs of early stage of hand eczema were registered. MWF from 3 trainee workshops were selected for predictive testing. MWF A was from the workshop with 36% of work-related skin changes (erythema, induration, flaking), MWF B from the workshop with 12% of skin changes, and MWF C from the workshop with 0% of skin changes. Exposure to irritants was found to be similar in the 3 trainee workshops.

Study Population

Fifteen healthy volunteer subjects, 6 male and 9 female without any skin diseases, entered the study after giving informed consent in accordance with the Helsinki declarations. The study had passed review by the Ethical Commission of the University Hospital Zurich. The age of the subjects was between 25 and 38 years with a mean age of 29.7. The study subjects were not allowed to use any detergents or creams on their backs during the days of investigation.

Test Substances

The water-based MWF are delivered by the producers as concentrates, which have to be diluted with water in the factory. We tested them at factories using concentrations of 3–5% diluted with water (pH 8.7–9.2).

Test Procedure

Two different tests were carried out on the same panel of subjects during October and November with the same 3 water-based MWF (A, B, C).

Test 1

This test model was based on the study of Hüner et al. [20] Application area was the paravertebral skin of the mid-back, and the test fields were randomised.

Test fields were treated with 0.05 ml of MWF applied with large Finn Chambers (12 mm diameter, filling volume 0.05 ml; Epitest Ltd., Hyrlä, Finland) and fixed with an overlapping sheet of Fixomull stretch tape (Beiersdorf, Hamburg, Germany). The chambers were removed after 24 h of exposure. 3 h after removal the test reactions were evaluated and new chambers were reapplied to the original sites, for a further 48 h, to induce a cumulative irritant reaction. Measurements were performed again after the 2nd exposure.

Test 2

Cumulative irritant contact dermatitis was induced using a repetitive irritation test for 2 weeks. Using the same MWF and kind of application as in test 1 the volunteers were treated from Monday to Friday in the first week and after the weekend from Monday to Thursday (in each case at the same time of day ± 1 h) for 6 h a day. Measurements were performed before the first application, on day 5 and again on day 12.

Measurements

Visual score (VS): 0 (none) to 5 (very severe with epidermal defects) as modified from Willis et al. [22]

Table 2. Test 1: mean values and SWM of the visual score, TEWL, and chromametry after single 24-hour patch test and repeated patch test (72 h)

24 h/72 h test		Visual score (0–5)			TEWL (g/m² h)			Chromametry (a*)		
		0 h	24 h	72 h	0 h	24 h	72 h	0 h	24 h	72 h
MWF A	mean	0.00	1.33	2.13	8.64	13.37	17.61	6.53	9.73	11.64
	SEM	0.00	0.18	0.27	0.87	1.25	2.11	0.48	0.78	0.96
MWF B	mean	0.00	1.07	1.40	8.97	10.67	12.38	6.34	8.83	9.59
	SEM	0.00	0.18	0.24	0.63	0.79	1.04	0.51	0.72	0.83
MWF C	mean	0.00	1.07	1.47	8.62	11.62	13.65	6.14	9.12	9.87
	SEM	0.00	0.18	0.16	0.77	1.06	0.95	0.55	0.63	0.69
Control	mean	0.00	0.07	0.20	8.12	8.74	8.75	6.12	6.56	6.90
(water)	SEM	0.00	0.06	0.11	0.58	0.59	0.50	0.52	0.53	0.43

Transepidermal water loss (TEWL) was measured with the Tewameter (Courage & Khazaka, Cologne, Germany). TEWL measurements were performed before application of the test substances at the beginning, after 24 h and after 72 h (test 1), and in test 2 by day 5 and day 12 following the recommendations for measurement of TEWL as described in detail by Pinnagoda et al. [23]

Measurements of skin colour were taken with the Chroma-Meter CR-200 (Minolta, Osaka, Japan) according to the recommendations of Elsner [24]. Each value is the average of 3 individual measurements.

Statistics

Statistical computations were performed with a statistical package (SPSS for the Macintosh, SPSS, Chicago, Il., USA) on an Apple Macintosh computer using an analysis of variance (one-way). All values are expressed as mean $\pm$ SEM. Pairs of groups are significantly different at the 0.050 level.

Results

The results of visual score, TEWL and chromametry in test 1 are shown in table 2. The mean baseline TEWL values and chromametry values were almost identical at the 4 test sites. After 24 h exposure, the visual score and the chromametry values of all MWF test sites increased significantly higher than controls. Even MWF C which was used in the workshop with 0% of work related skin changes showed irritant potential. The TEWL was significantly different between control and MWF A and between control and MWF C (table 4). In the visual score, MWF B and MWF C had the same value. After

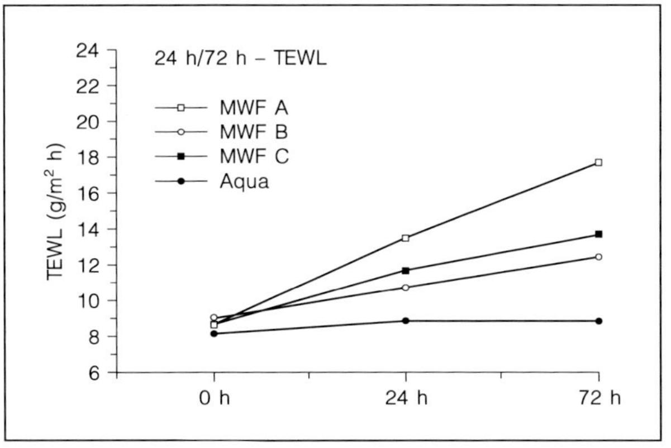

Fig. 1. Test 1: The effect of different MWF in TEWL after a single 24-hour patch test and repeated patch test (72 h). Results are given as mean. The following irritancy ranking of test substances is seen after 24 and 72 h: MWF A > MWF C > MWF B > water.

Table 3. Test 2: mean values and SEM of the visual score, TEWL, and chromametry after 5 and 12 days' repeated patch test

5 days/12 days test		Visual score (0–5)			TEWL (g/m^2 h)			Chromametry (a*)		
		day 0	day 5	day 12	day 0	day 5	day 12	day 0	day 5	day 12
MWF A	mean	0.00	0.46	1.06	8.73	13.56	16.77	6.28	7.37	7.49
	SEM	0.00	0.13	0.18	0.66	1.24	1.79	0.57	0.43	0.69
MWF B	mean	0.00	0.20	0.47	8.47	11.01	11.35	6.18	6.54	6.66
	SEM	0.00	0.10	0.13	0.63	0.86	0.86	0.54	0.46	0.39
MWF C	mean	0.00	0.27	0.60	8.91	12.53	14.34	6.38	7.06	7.07
	SEM	0.00	0.12	0.16	1.03	0.94	1.49	0.55	0.56	0.60
Control	mean	0.00	0.00	0.06	8.92	8.98	9.54	6.28	6.38	6.46
(water)	SEM	0.00	0.00	0.06	0.67	0.55	0.56	0.53	0.52	0.50

the 72 h exposure, we observed a further increase for all parameters which were also significantly higher than those treated with water. The ranking for the test substances after 24 and 72 h was MWF A > MWF C > MWF B for the visual score, the TEWL and the chromametry values. Figure 1 shows the mean TEWL of test sites over the 72-hour study period.

The means and SEM of visual score, TEWL and chromametry in test 2 are shown in table 3. As observed in test 1 MWF A caused the highest increase

Table 4. Discriminative power of the visual score, TEWL, and chromametry in the two test models

		24 h/72 h test		5 days/12 days test
Visual score	24 h	water MWF B MWF C MWF A	5 days	water MWF B MWF C MWF A
	72 h	water MWF B MWF C MWF A	12 days	water MWF B MWF C MWF A
TEWL	24 h	water MWF B MWF C MWF A	5 days	water MWF B MWF C MWF A
	72 h	water MWF B MWF C MWF A	12 days	water MWF B MWF C MWF A
Chromametry	24 h	water MWF B MWF C MWF A	5 days	water MWF B MWF C MWF A no significant differences
	72 h	water MWF B MWF C MWF A	12 days	water MWF B MWF C MWF A no significant differences

The substances are ordered with respect to their means. Substances which are significantly different at the 0.050 level are connected by underlining.

in TEWL which was nearly the same as in the 24 h/72 h model whereas all values of visual score and chromametry were much lower in test 2 than in the 72-hour study period. We performed the same ranking for the test substances as in test 1. The analysis of variance in this test model showed a worse differentiation of the substances, e.g. fewer significant differences were observed at the 0.050 level (table 4). Figure 2 shows the mean TEWL of test sites over the 12-day study period.

Discussion

In both test models we observed an increase in visual score, TEWL, and chromametry for all MWF tested compared with water used as control. The same irritancy ranking of the substances was detected. Although the 2-week exposure with repetitive and cumulative contact with MWFs seems to be

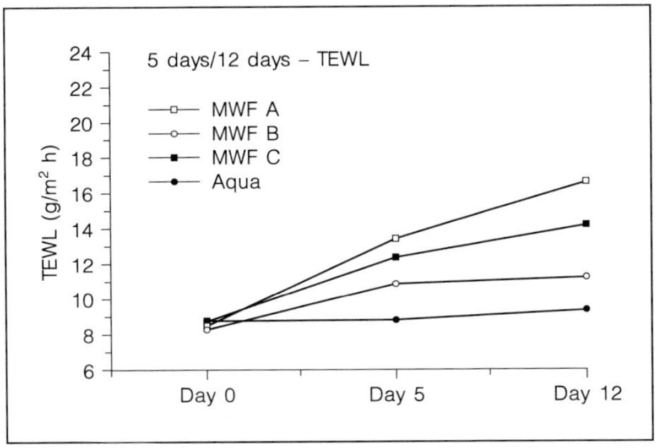

Fig. 2. Test 2: The effect of different MWF in TEWL after 5 and 12 days' repeated patch test. Results are given as mean. The following irritancy ranking of test substances is seen after 24 and 72 h: MWF A > MWF C > MWF B > water.

nearer to real-life exposure than the short-time model, the analysis of variance (one-way) showed a better differentiation of the MWF in the single 24-hour patch test with repeated application to 72 h in VS, TEWL and chromametry than the other model. After 72 h of occlusive MWF exposure the visual score shows the same or a better differentiation in substances than the measurements of TEWL and chromametry. Therefore, it might be argued that bioengineering techniques such as TEWL and chromametry are not necessary for the predictive testing of MWF irritancy. However, clinical examinations like the visual score are a subjective and quantitative assessment and depend on the examiner in contrast to TEWL and chromametry that provide objective and qualitative data.

Furthermore, test model 2 showed that measurement of TEWL provides sensitive information about epidermal barrier impairment by MWF, before this becomes detectable by the visual score especially if the MWF causes only a weak reaction. Though the chromametry characterises a different aspect of irritation than the TEWL, it provided no better differentiation between the MWF. Considering the shorter application time and the better discrimination of irritancy we prefer the first model as a routine procedure for the predictive testing of MWF irritancy and propose the visual score and the TEWL for measurements.

So far there has been no conclusive evidence that results from predictive testing of MWF are applicable to real working conditions. A randomised, double-blind clinical study would be necessary to provide this kind of data.

This has never been performed, and it does not seem to be practicable. Hüner et al. [20] reported that a switch from the 2 most irritant MWFs to a less irritant MWF in their test resulted in a reduction of irritant reactions in a metalworking factory. However, the authors do not give more specific information on this kind of open intervention.

Alternatively, epidemiological data may be compared with product testing under experimental conditions, as was the case in our study. To our knowledge, no comparable data have been published yet. Our experimental results partially confirm the data of PROMETES. Workers who were exposed to MWF A which showed the highest increase in VS, TEWL and chromametry in both tests developed ICD more often than those exposed to MWF B and MWF C.

In both test models the ranking between the MWF with no development of ICD in the workshop (C) and the MWF with 12% of ICD (B) was in reverse order to the epidemiological data. A reason for this finding could be that various confounders like the disposition to atopy, the extent of MWF exposure or the use of after-work emollients or more or less irritating cleaning products in the factories may influence the outcome even if the irritancy potential of the MWF is low. Still, a coarse classification of MWF seems to be possible using the shown predictive tests while the assessment of mild irritating products remains problematic.

Because of the variable prognosis of contact dermatitis in metalworkers [25–28], prevention and early intervention in irritant dermatitis is of utmost importance. Protection by barrier creams is not convincing [17, 29], and gloves carry the risk of accidents. We propose that the selection of MWF based on the results of a standardized predictive test as reported in this study may significantly reduce skin problems in metalworkers.

References

1 De Boer EM, van Ketel WG, Bruynzeel DP: Dermatoses in metalworkers. I. Irritant contact dermatitis. Contact Dermatitis 1989;20:212–218.

2 Rycroft RJG: Soluble oil dermatitis. Clin Exp Dermatol 1981;6:229–234.

3 Foulds IS, Kohn D: Dermatitis from metalworking fluids. Clin Exp Dermatol 1990;15:157–162.

4 Alomar A, Conde-Salazar L, Romaguera C: Occupational dermatoses from cutting oils. Contact Dermatitis 1985;12:129–138.

5 Itschner L, Hinnen U, Elsner P: Skin risk assessment of metalworking fluids: A survey among Swiss suppliers. Allergologie 1995;18:466.

6 Grattan CEH, English JSC, Foulds IS, Rycroft RJG: Cutting fluid dermatitis. Contact Dermatitis 1989;20:372–376.

7 De Boer EM, van Ketel WG, Bruynzeel DP: Dermatoses in metalworkers. II. Allergic contact dermatitis. Contact Dermatitis 1989;20:280–286.

8 Hodgson G: Eczemas associated with lubricants and metalworking fluids. Dermatol Dig 1976; October:11–15.

9 Fisher AA: Allergic contact dermatitis of the hands due to industrial oils and fluids. Cutis 1979; 23:131–142.
10 Alomar A: Occupational skin disease from cutting fluids. Dermatol Clin 1994;12:537–546.
11 Goh CL, Yuen R: A study of occupational skin disease in the metal industry (1986-1990). Ann Acad Med Singapore 1994;23:639–344.
12 Goh CL, Gan SL: The incidence of cutting fluid dermatitis among metalworkers in a metal fabrication factory: A prospective study. Contact Dermatitis 1994;31:111–115.
13 Diepgen T, Schmidt A, Schmidt M, Fartasch M: Demographic and legal characteristics of occupational skin diseases. Allergologie 1994;17:84–89.
14 Price D, White J, English J, Rycroft RJG: Soluble oil dermatitis. A review. J Soc Occup Med 1989; 39:93–98.
15 Hinnen U, Elsner P: PROMETES: A 3-year follow-up study in metalworker trainees: Preliminary results. Allergologie 1995;18:455–456.
16 Patrick E, Maibach HI: Predictive assays: Animal and man, and in vitro and in vivo; in Rycroft RJG, Menné T, Frosch PJ (eds): Textbook of Contact Dermatitis. Berlin, Springer, 1992, pp 706–740.
17 Goh CL: Cutting oil dermatitis on guinea pig skin. I. Cutting oil dermatitis and barrier cream. Contact Dermatitis 1991;24:16–21.
18 Goh CL: Cutting oil dermatitis on guinea pig skin. II. Emollient creams and cutting oil dermatitis. Contact Dermatitis 1991;24:81–85.
19 de Boer EM, Scholten RJPM, van Ketel WG, Bruynzeel DP: The irritancy of metalworker fluids: A laser Doppler flowmetry study. Contact Dermatitis 1990;22:86–94.
20 Hüner A, Fartasch M, Hornstein OP, Diepgen TL: The irritant effect of different metalworking fluids. Contact Dermatitis 1994;31:220–225.
21 Coenraads PJ, Foo SC, Phoon WO, Lun KC: Dermatitis in small-scale metal industries. Contact Dermatitis 1985;12:155–160.
22 Willis CM, Stephens JM, Wilkinson JD: Experimentally-induced irritant contact dermatitis. Contact Dermatitis 1988;18:20–24.
23 Pinnagoda J, Tupker RA, Agner T, Serup J. Guidelines for transepidermal water loss (TEWL) measurement. Report Standardization Group Eur Soc Contact Dermatitis. Contact Dermatitis 1990;22:164–178.
24 Elsner P: Chromametry Hardware, measuring principles and standardization of measurements, in: Beradesca E, Elsner P, Maibach HI (eds): Handbooks of Skin Bioengineering. Cutaneous Blood Flow and Erythema. Boca Raton, CRC Press, 1994, pp 347–352.
25 Pryce DW, Irvine D, English JSC, Rycroft RJG: What happens to patients with soluble-oil dermatitis? Br J Dermatol 1989;(suppl 34):27–28.
26 Johnson ML, Wilson HTH: Oil dermatitis: An enquiry into its prognosis. Br J Ind Med 1971;28: 122–125.
27 Mackey SA, Marks JG: Dermatitis in machinists: A retrospective study. Am J Contact Dermatitis 1993;4:22–26.
28 Grattan CEH, Foulds IS: Outcome of investigation of cutting fluid dermatitis. Contact Dermatitis 1989;20:377–378.
29 Goh CL, Gan SL: Efficacies of a barrier cream and an afterwork emollient cream against cutting fluid dermatitis in metalworkers: A prospective study. Contact Dermatitis 1994;31:176–180.

Prof. Dr. Peter Elsner, University of Zurich, Gloriastrasse 31, CH–8091 Zurich (Switzerland)

Elsner P, Lachapelle JM, Wahlberg JE, Maibach HI (eds): Prevention of Contact Dermatitis. Curr Probl Dermatol. Basel, Karger, 1996, vol 25, pp 116–122

Prevention of Hand Eczema in Atopics

Birgitta Meding

Division of Occupational Dermatology, National Institute for Working Life and Department of Occupational Dermatology, Karolinska Hospital, Solna, Sweden

Prevalence of Atopic Dermatitis

Atopic dermatitis is a common skin disease. A cumulative incidence of 12% was reported by Åberg et al. [1] in Swedish children aged 7–14 in 1989. Recent studies present even higher figures. One example is the United Kingdom study by Kay et al. [2], in which a lifetime occurrence of 20% was found in children aged 3–11 years. An increasing prevalence has been documented during the past few decades. Before 1960 about 2–3% of children had atopic dermatitis. For those born in the 1960s, 4–8% was the prevalence found in several studies, and later 10–20% has been reported [3–8]. The causes of the increasing prevalence are not clear. The disposition for atopy is hereditary but genetic changes of this magnitude in a few decades are improbable. It has been speculated that environmental factors are responsible for activating latent disease but it has not been possible to define what these factors are. Changes in the host defence have also been discussed and the role of fewer parasitic infections in the Western industrialized countries might be of importance.

Atopic Dermatitis and Hand Eczema

In several studies a correlation between atopic dermatitis and hand eczema in adult life has been shown. At the beginning of the 1980s in Stockholm, Rystedt [9] followed-up 955 persons with moderate and severe atopic dermatitis in childhood. She found that 48–60% had developed hand eczema after the age of 15. A similar study was later presented from Finland. Here

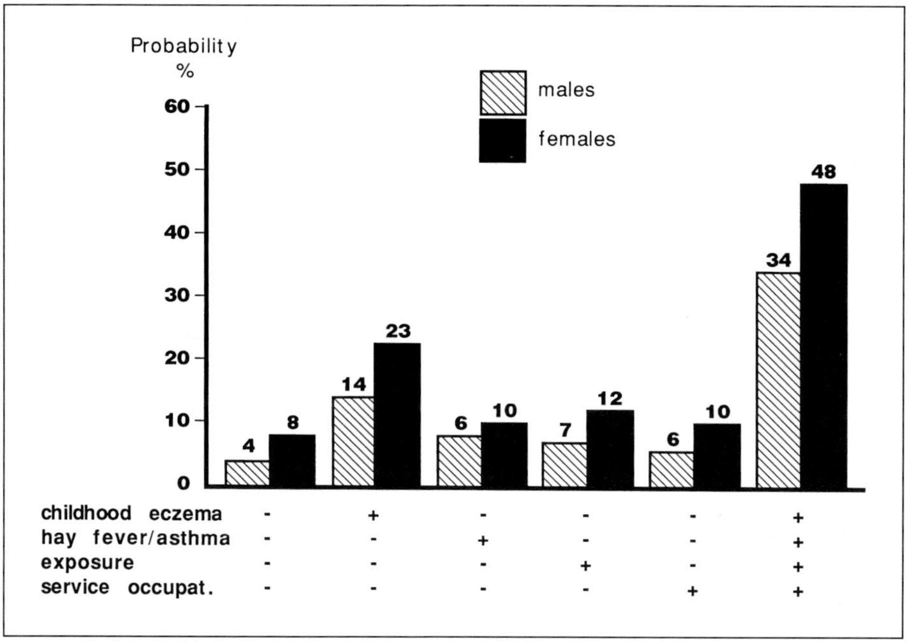

Fig. 1. Examples of the estimated probability of developing hand eczema in a 12-month period in relation to gender, childhood eczema, asthma/hay fever, occupational exposure and service occupation. [From Contact Dermatitis 1990;23:154–161, with permission.]

Lammintausta and Kalimo [10] found at follow-up that patients with severe and moderate atopic dermatitis during their teens had a 2-year period prevalence of hand eczema of 54–71% and those with mild atopic dermatitis about 40%. The prognosis for atopics in some occupations has been studied. Nilsson et al. [11], in Sweden, followed newly employed hospital workers prospectively for 20 months. They found that the occurrence of hand eczema during the follow-up time was about 60% in wet work for those with atopic dermatitis. The odds of developing hand eczema was increased almost 3 times for persons with a history of atopic dermatitis in both wet and dry hospital work. In a study at Turku Hospital, Finland, Lammintausta and Kalimo [12] also found that 65% of persons with a history of atopic dermatitis and occupied in wet hospital work had hand eczema. In a prevalence study in the general population of Gothenburg, Sweden, a threefold increase in hand eczema prevalence was found in individuals with a history of childhood dermatitis [13]. The results were based on answers to a questionnaire from 16,584 randomly selected individuals aged 20–65 years. In a multivariate stepwise logistic regression analysis, it was found that childhood eczema was the most important predictor for hand eczema, more important than occupational exposure. In figure 1, calculations based on results from the study illustrate the risk of hand eczema in a 1-year period in relation to atopy, occupational exposure and gender. The single most important parameter was childhood eczema and the combination of risk factors gave an estimated risk for males of 34% and for females 48%.

Occupational Skin Disease

Hand eczema is the most common occupational skin disease making up about 90% of the cases. In Sweden all reports of occupational disease are sent to the Occupational Injury Information Division at the National Board of Occupational Safety and Health in Stockholm. Individuals younger than 25 years report skin disease from work twice as often as older people, and females report more frequently than males. In a recent investigation of the medical basis for 655 cases of reported occupational skin disease it was found that a history of atopic dermatitis was documented in the medical reports of 40% of the cases aged 16–24 years compared to 17% in those aged 25–64 years ($p < 0.001$) [Meding, to be publ.]. This illustrates that young atopics get skin problems when entering working life, and agrees with earlier reports on occupational dermatoses [14, 15].

Increasing Prevalence of Hand Eczema?

Considering the strong correlation between atopic dermatitis and hand eczema, the increasing occurrence of atopic dermatitis in the population can be expected to lead to an increased number of adults with hand eczema. A comparison of the hand eczema prevalence in Sweden in the 1980s and 1960s is possible and indicates such a tendency. In Gothenburg the point prevalence of hand eczema in the general population was estimated to be about 5% at the beginning of the 1980s [16]. Twenty years earlier Agrup [17] found a prevalence of 2–3% in the south of Sweden. Comparing the diagnoses in the two studies shows that the major difference in prevalence rates concerns atopic hand eczema [18]. Whether the increasing atopy trend will continue is impossible to predict. In some recent studies on the occurrence of atopic dermatitis the conclusion is that the increase in prevalence seems to have retarded [19].

Risk Exposure

It has been discussed whether there are certain exogenous factors that trigger the hand eczema in atopics. It seems that in young atopics it often tends to appear shortly after entering working life. In Rystedt's [9] follow-up study, the prevalence was higher in occupations with skin irritant exposure and it was also found that such exposure gave rise to more severe dermatitis. In a Finnish study the occupational exposure in relation to the course of an atopic skin disease was investigated by Lammintausta and Kalimo [10]. They found an evident correlation between hand eczema in atopic patients and occupational exposure. Ninety percent of the atopic patients developed hand eczema if they had occupational skin irritant exposure for 2 h or more daily. With little or no corresponding exposure, only 50% had hand eczema.

Risk Occupations

Regarding a possible rationale for vocational guidance to atopics there is no unanimous answer to the question of whether young persons with atopic dermatitis should avoid certain occupations. The choice of occupation is perhaps of universal importance and many different factors are to be considered. An occupation that suits the talents and interests of the individual is crucial, and staying healthy and able to continue in one's job is also important. Some dermatologists do not recommend a restrictive occupational counselling policy but suggest early information on the nature of the skin disease and on skin protection [10]. Others are of the opinion that the risk levels in different occupations should also be considered [20]. However, all young persons with atopic dermatitis should get enough knowledge about their skin disease to be aware of the increased risk of hand eczema. It is important that the higher risk in occupations with skin irritant exposure, and the prognosis for remaining in the occupation, are considered together with other important factors for the choice of occupation.

In Rystedt's study the main risk occupations for hand eczema among atopics were food handling, hairdressing, nursing, laboratory and domestic work, cleaning, building and metalwork [9]. From the register of the Swedish Information System on Occupational Injuries, high-risk occupations have been calculated related to the number of individuals employed in the occupations [21]. For skin disease, which is hand eczema in 90% of the cases, the number-one risk occupation was hairdresser with a rate ratio (SIR) of 5.4 followed by machinery fitter, cook, dental nurse, machine-tool operator, cleaner, kitchen maid and assistant nurse (fig. 2).

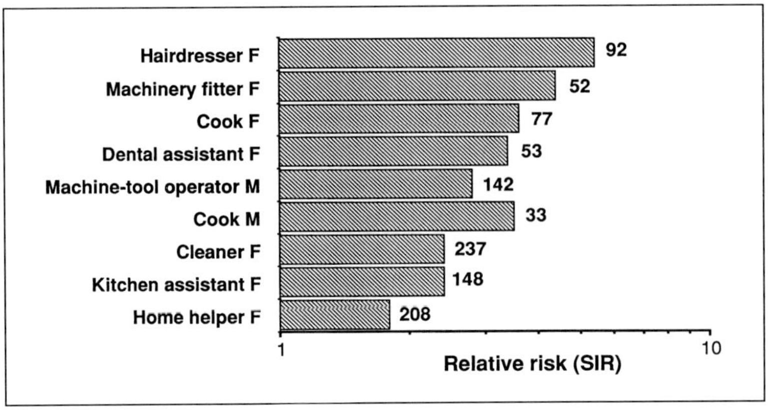

Fig. 2. High-risk occupations for occupational skin disease in Sweden 1990–1991 expressed as relative risk. Number of cases reported to the Information System on Occupational Injuries above the bars. Employment information obtained from census (FoB 90).

A low proportion of atopics in some occupations can represent a hint that the occupation is unsuitable for atopics and has been avoided or abandoned by such people. In the Gothenburg hand eczema study there was a significantly smaller proportion of persons with a history of childhood eczema in production work and service work [13].

Risk Individuals

The hand eczema risk is not identical for all atopics. Rystedt [20] performed a multivariate analysis to estimate predictors for hand eczema. The results made it possible to divide at-risk individuals into high-, medium-, and low-risk individuals. The extreme high-risk individual had hand eczema already in childhood, persistent body eczema in adult life and persistently dry and itching skin. With these strong predictors the risk of hand eczema in adult life was 90% in occupations with skin irritant exposure and 81% in other occupations. The corresponding figure for those without these strong predictors was 9%.

Skin Hygiene and Protection

One possible way to prevent hand eczema is by skin hygiene and skin protection. The effect of such procedures in the occupational setting has not been investigated much. Skin-care products, e.g. emollients, and protective gloves are usually recommended to the hand eczema patient. The effect of such measures on the induction, course and prognosis of hand eczema in different occupational situations and in relation to different types and levels of exposure is largely unknown. There is a need for large enough and carefully designed intervention studies to estimate the effects of such measures to be able to design effective preventive programs for a number of occupational demands.

Prognosis of Atopic Hand Eczema

The prognosis of atopic hand eczema has been investigated in some studies. In the Gothenburg hand eczema study a number of parameters reflecting the severity of the eczema were compared for different types of hand eczema. It seemed that atopic hand eczema was a more widespread and long-standing disease [22]. This was a cross-sectional study and thus observations over time were not possible. Lammintausta et al. [23] found atopic dermatitis in a considerable number of the most chronic hand eczema cases among hospital workers. Shmunes and Keil [14] concluded that the role of atopy figured dramatically among the most serious cases of occupational dermatoses in South Carolina. A poor prognosis for the healing of hand eczema in atopics has also been found in several other studies [15, 24, 25].

Conclusions

Atopic hand eczema is a challenge for the dermatologist. Considering the probably increasing prevalence, preventive measures are urgent. To be able to effectively prevent the disease, knowledge of risk factors is a prerequisite. Of primary importance in the preventive process is to realize the strong correlation between atopic dermatitis and hand eczema. Risk factors have to be identified and their relative importance investigated. The effect of separate interventions should be estimated. There is great need for further research about atopic hand eczema to obtain a solid basis for the construction of preventive programs.

References

1 Åberg N, Engström I, Lindberg U: Allergic diseases in Swedish school children. Acta Paediatr Scand 1989;78:246–252.

2 Kay J, Gawkrodger DJ, Mortimer MJ, Jaron AG: The prevalence of childhood atopic eczema in a general population. J Am Acad Dermatol 1994;30:35–39.

3 Taylor B, Wadsworth J, Wadsworth M, Peckham C: Changes in the reported prevalence of childhood eczema since the 1939–1945 war. Lancet 1984;i:1255–1257.

4 Burr ML, Butland BK, King S, Vaughan-Williams E: Changes in asthma prevalence: Two surveys 15 years apart. Arch Dis Child 1989;64:1452–1456.

5 Schultz Larsen F, Hanifin JM: Secular change in the occurrence of atopic dermatitis. Acta Derm Venereol 1992;(suppl 176):7–12.

6 Williams HC: Is the prevalence of atopic dermatitis increasing? Clin Exp Dermatol 1992;17:385–391.

7 Ninan TK, Russell G: Respiratory symptoms and atopy in Aberdeen schoolchildren: Evidence from two surveys 25 years apart. BMJ 1992;304:873–875.

8 Dotterud L-K, Kvammen B, Bolle R, Falk ES: A survey of atopic diseases among school children in Sør-Varanger community: Possible effects of subarctic climate and industrial pollution from Russia. Acta Derm Venereol 1994;74:124–128.

9 Rystedt I: Work-related hand eczema in atopics. Contact Dermatitis 1985;12:164–171.

10 Lammintausta K, Kalimo K: Does a patient's occupation influence the course of atopic dermatitis? Acta Derm Venereol 1993;73:119–122.

11 Nilsson E, Mikaelsson B, Andersson S: Atopy, occupation and domestic work as risk factors for hand eczema in hospital workers. Contact Dermatitis 1985;13:216–233.

12 Lammintausta K, Kalimo K: Atopy and hand dermatitis in hospital wet work. Contact Dermatitis 1981;7:301–308.

13 Meding B, Swanbeck G: Predictive factors for hand eczema. Contact Dermatitis 1990;23:154–161.

14 Shmunes E, Keil J: The role of atopy in occupational dermatoses. Contact Dermatitis 1984;11: 174–178.

15 Rystedt I: Atopic background in patients with occupational hand eczema. Contact Dermatitis 1985; 12:247–254.

16 Meding B, Swanbeck G: Prevalence of hand eczema in an industrial city. Br J Dermatol 1987;116: 627–634.

17 Agrup G: Hand eczema and other hand dermatoses in South Sweden. Acta Derm Venereol 1969; (suppl 61):22–27.

18 Meding B, Swanbeck G: Epidemiology of different types of hand eczema. Acta Derm Venereol 1989;69:227–233.

19 Varjonen E, Kalimo K, Lammintausta K, Tero P: Prevalence of atopic disorders among adolescents in Turku, Finland. Allergy 1992;47:243–248.

20 Rystedt I: Hand eczema and long-term prognosis in atopic dermatitis; thesis. Stockholm, Karolinska Institute, 1985.

21 Hedlin M, Bengtsson B, Norell M, Malker H: Anmälda hudsjukdomar i arbetslivet. Arbetarskyddsstyrelsen, Solna, Sweden, Rapport 1994; 10.

22 Meding B: Epidemiology of hand eczema in an industrial city. Acta Derm Venereol 1990;(suppl 153): 26–29.

23 Lammintausta K, Kalimo K, Aantaa S: Course of hand dermatitis in hospital workers. Contact Dermatitis 1982;8:327–332.

24 Nilsson E, Bäck O: The importance of anamnestic information of atopy, metal dermatitis and earlier hand eczema for the development of hand dermatitis in women in wet hospital work. Acta Derm Venereol 1986;66:45–50.

25 Rosen RH, Freeman S: Prognosis of occupational contact dermatitis in New South Wales, Australia. Contact Dermatitis 1993;29:88–93.

Birgitta Meding, MD, Division of Occupational Dermatology, National Institute for Working Life, S–171 84 Solna (Sweden)

Elsner P, Lachapelle JM, Wahlberg JE, Maibach HI (eds): Prevention of Contact Dermatitis. Curr Probl Dermatol. Basel, Karger, 1996, vol 25, pp 123–132

Risk-Group-Related Prevention of Hand Eczema at the Workplace

Ulrich Funke[a], *Thomas L. Diepgen*[b], *Manigé Fartasch*[b]

[a] Gesundheitswesen AUDI AG, Ingolstadt and
[b] Department of Dermatology, University of Erlangen-Nuremberg, Germany

One of the major principles of occupational medicine is the identification of risk groups for work-related diseases and then to prevent them by reducing the risks at the workplace and by special occupational medical care. Irritant contact dermatitis (ICD) is the most important work-related skin disease. Within the last 10 years the knowlege of ICD has expanded considerably as a result of dermatologic research, close cooperation of dermatologists and occupational physicians and especially as a result of population-based epidemiologic studies. This new knowledge and the resulting adjusted tools for prevention of ICD also offer new possibilities to enforce prevention of ICD by more intense participation of the subjects themselves in preventive measures at the workplace. Finally new structures of the organization of the work, such as work in production teams, can be used successfully for this purpose.

High-Risk Groups for Hand Eczema

For the identification of risk groups for hand eczema (HE) some preliminary results of an ongoing (1990–1998) prospective cohort study are given, which is performed in close long-term cooperation with the Department of Dermatology of the University of Erlangen-Nuremberg [1]. 2,100 apprentices at AUDI AG in Ingolstadt and Neckarsulm were examined before the start, after the first year and at the end of their apprenticeships. The first examinations were performed before the start of the apprenticeship by specially trained occupational physicians as part of the usual preemployment examinations. At this time the subjects were not aware of a study situation. There was no preemployment selection in respect of skin history by occupational physicians (participants did not know this). Recorded parameters were skin history, atopic features [2] and domestic skin hazards. The second and third examinations were performed by dermatologists. Additional parameters like use of barrier creams and occupational irritants, e.g. wet work, were evaluated at the third examination. The diagnosis of hand eczema (outcome variable) was set up by dermatologists according to the following definition: reported skin problems (like redness, itching and scaling) during the apprenticeship with the localisation at the hands and/or forearms. The diagnosis was supported by standardized documentations of eczematous lesions at the hands and forearms during the apprenticeship in the department of occupational medicine. Mycosis or other not job-related eczema were excluded.

Currently, 2,115 1st examinations, 1,597 2nd and 727 3rd examinations have been performed. 79% of the apprentices were male and 21% female. No examination was yet refused by the apprentices. The drop out rate was 5.9% within the first year and 9.9% within the whole apprenticeship. Actual follow-up (set date 31.08.95) was 98.8%, because 83% of the drop outs answered a questionnaire with items about HE before they left the company.

Predisposing factors, exposure to irritants at the workplace, domestic skin hazards and the use of barrier creams are the most interesting factors in the prevention of work-related HE. To calculate distributions and relative risks for HE of these parameters, the results of 1,597 2nd examinations and 727 3rd examinations linked with the 1st examinations were evaluated.

The overall 1-year incidence rate of HE was 6.3% and the 3-year incidence rate was 12.9%. Women had a significantly elevated HE risk (9.2%) compared to men (5.6%) within a 1-year period (3-year incidence rates: females: 18.0%; males: 11.6%). Of the other predisposing factors a history of HE, atopic eczema (AE) and dyshidrosis had the highest relative risks (RR) for HE in the observed periods of 1 and 3 years (fig. 1). All other parameters and especially a personal or family history of respiratory atopy had only a moderate association with HE. For preventive measures and individual medical advice the predictive values for HE of the different risk factors are important. Taking into account moderate exposures to irritants at the workplace a history of HE, AE and dyshidrosis were associated with predictive values for HE between 40 and 24% within a 1-year period and between 45 and 40% within a 3-year period. Predictive values of all other parameters were below 20%.

Wet work as a widespread summarizing factor of exposure to irritants at the workplace raises the ratio of HE significantly (RR 1.9), only when it exceeds 3 h a day within a 3-year period (fig. 2). Other often discussed confounders for HE are domestic exposures to irritants [3]. Males and females had their own

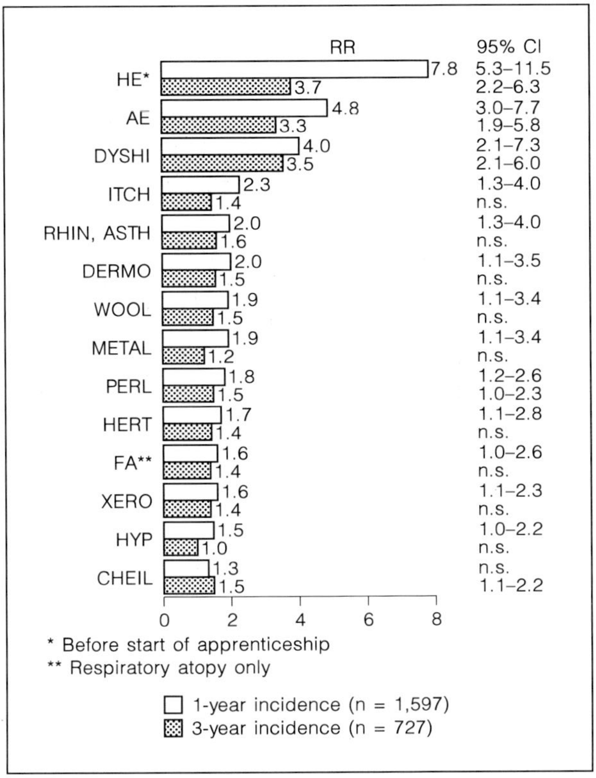

Fig. 1. Parameters with significant high RR for HE.

typical domestic exposures to different irritants. Continuously (daily before and after the 1st year of apprenticeship) washing of dishes performed by 22.3% of the young women causes no increased risk for HE (RR: 1.0; 95% CI: 0.5–2.3) within the first year of apprenticeship. On the other hand, handicraft work and car repair performed continuously daily-weekly by 8.0% of the young men was associated with a RR for HE of 2.1 (1.2–3.9) and house building performed continuously daily-weekly (2.3%) with a RR for HE of 4.0 (1.9–8.4).

The regular use of barrier creams may reduce the risk of HE, but HE itself seems to be the most important factor for the use of barrier creams. Therefore the evaluation of the effectiveness of barrier creams in the prevention of HE cannot be analyzed in this epidemiologic study. But even in high-risk groups the use of barrier creams is not sufficient. In the metalwork

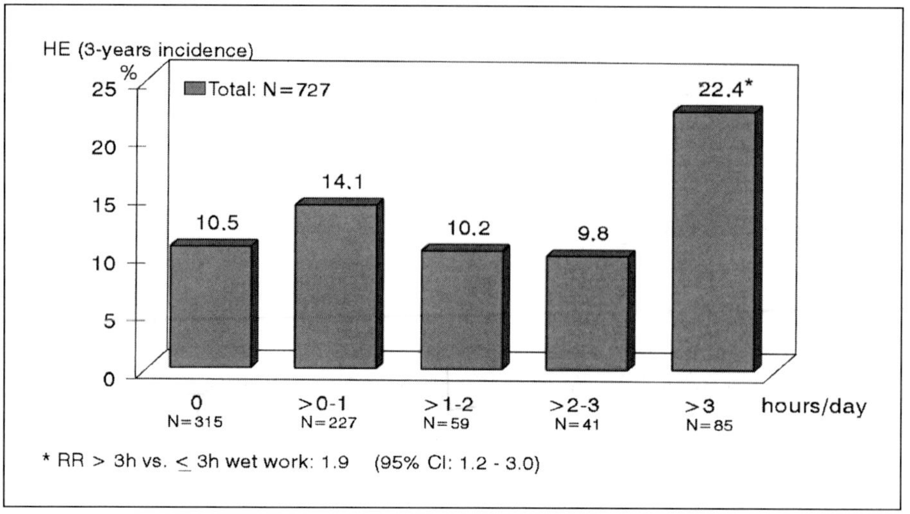

Fig. 2. HE and wet work at the workplace. Observed period: 3 years.

apprenticeship only 19.3% of apprentices with HE in the last year and only 7.5% without HE used the free available barrier creams twice a day or more (fig. 3).

In summarizing the results, predisposing factors like history of HE, AE and dyshidrosis are the most relevant for HE within a short time period and for moderate exposure to irritants at the workplace. Female gender is associated with an elevated HE risk unaffected by domestic hazards. Exposure to wet work becomes relevant for HE if it exceeds several hours a day for some years. Frequency and time of exposure to some domestic hazards have to be recorded as they may cause HE in a considerable part of the population. It is remarkable that the relevant domestic risk factors result from primary occupational activities, which were performed without any occupational medical care.

Special Periodical Medical Examinations and Risk Groups for Hand Eczema

Looking at the actual setting in prevention of ICD with some limitations, it is possible to predict the individual HE risk in respect of predisposing factors, occupational and domestic exposure to irritants. Even the high-risk

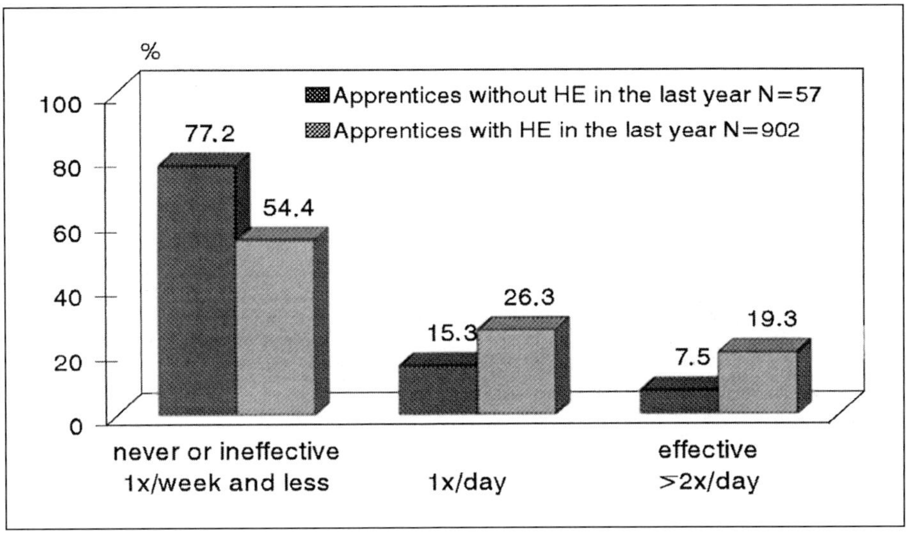

Fig. 3. Use of barrier creams in metalwork apprenticeship.

groups for ICD do not use barrier creams sufficiently. This indicates that the risk groups have no sufficient knowledge regarding their higher risk of developing HE and so they probably will not perform other measures of skin protection like use of protective gloves or generally avoid skin contact with irritants whenever possible. In this situation, special periodical medical examinations are an effective preventive tool.

Special periodical medical examinations not only include identification of high-risk groups and early diagnosis of occupational skin diseases (OSD) but also individual advice to minimize skin contact with irritants/allergens and appropriate use of protection equipment and barrier creams. Job selection according to individual risk of OSD remains necessary only for a minority of subjects with extreme susceptibility of the skin and jobs with long-term unavoidable exposures to irritants or subjects with clinically relevant and really job-relevant allergies.

All subjects with relevant exposures to irritants at the workplace (for example with 2 h of wet work a day and more) then ought to be included in special periodical medical examinations. The German Berufsgenossenschaften (professional associations having the liability for industrial safety and insurance) have just revised their instructions for special periodical medical examinations for the prevention of OSD. In these new instructions risk groups for OSD are defined as follows (examples):

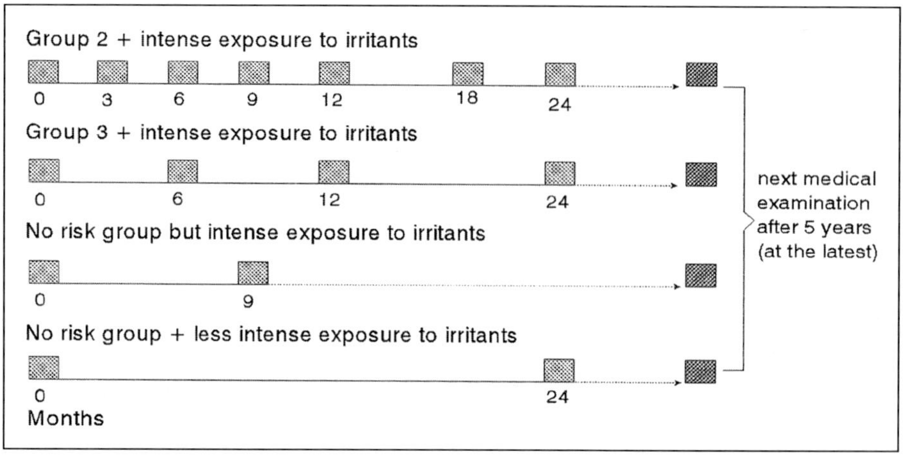

Fig. 4. Risk group and exposure-related intervals of periodical medical examinations (examples).

Group 1 (very high risk):	AE (severe) + HE (long-lasting or recurring), HE (severe + chronical or recurring) ...
Group 2 (high risk):	AE (without HE), dishydrosis ...
Group 3 (moderate risk):	Wool intolerance, itch when sweating, xerosis, ...

To minimize the requirement of exclusion from jobs with exposures to irritants, which remains relevant for group 1 (with very high risk for OSD), all other subjects were included in the periodical examinations. The intervals of examinations were then adjusted for risk group and degree of exposure. Subjects of group 2 with intense exposure to irritants like hairdressers will then be examined every 3 months within the first year and subjects without predisposing factors and only a less intense exposure to irritants at the workplace may be seen by the doctor after 2 years (fig. 4). This concept promises a high efficiency because it concentrates all activities on a valid description of risk groups. The definitions of the risk groups are in quite good accordance with the results of our epidemiological study.

Self-Assessment of Risk of Hand Eczema, Work In Production Teams and Prevention

Special periodical medical examinations will trigger and enforce avoidance of exposure to irritants and proper use of protective equipment and barrier creams. For the continuous stabilization of risk-adapted behavior on the one hand individual awareness of risk, and communication and behavior patterns within the production teams on the other, are decisive.

Therefore, a skin protection campaign including a questionnaire for the self-assessment of HE risk was started in the department of motor and chassis parts manufacturing. The manufacturing processes are turning, milling, drilling and assembly of the engine and the complete power train. 40% of the 2,236 production workers are included in special periodical medical examinations. Two years previously, the organisation of the work had changed completely in the production and now all workers are integrated into 237 production teams.

As a basis for the skin protection campaign a skin protection brochure was developed. The contents of this brochure were 4 questions for the self-assessment of HE risk, deriving from preliminary results of the prospective cohort study: (1) hand or forearm eczema; (2) flexural eczema; (3) hay fever, allergic asthma or allergic conjunctivitis, and itch when sweating.

Other questions concerned the use of barrier creams at the workplace and at home. Additionally, some risk groups and exposure-to-irritant-related advice for skin protection and medical care were given. And, finally, a small competition was included.

The implementation of the campaign was based on the team leaders as disseminators. All team leaders were trained about the aims, objectives and organisation of the campaign. Then each team leader distributed the brochures in his production team and the questions were discussed and answered at regular team meetings. The return of the questionnaire part of the brochure was again organized by the team leaders and participation of 94% (2,102/2,236) was reached this way.

For the evaluation of the validity of self-assessment of HE risk reported frequencies of parameters and their association to HE are relevant. The frequencies of flexural eczema (7.9%), hay fever (14.2%) and itch when sweating (14.6%) agreed quite well with the results of the cohort study and other population-based studies [4, 5]. The frequency of HE (26.5%) was plausible too as we asked for a lifelong history of HE; the median age in that sample was 34 years. In figure 5, the relative risks and their 95% confidence intervals of HE (lifelong history) for the three other parameters of the questionnaire were calculated. The results were nearly the same as in the 3-year incidence analysis of the cohort study (fig. 1) and the confidence intervals were, as a result of the large sample, rather small.

Although the use of barrier creams in motor and chassis parts manufacturing was rather more intense than in metalworkers undergoing an apprenticeship, the structure of the results was the same: 48.2% of the workers with and

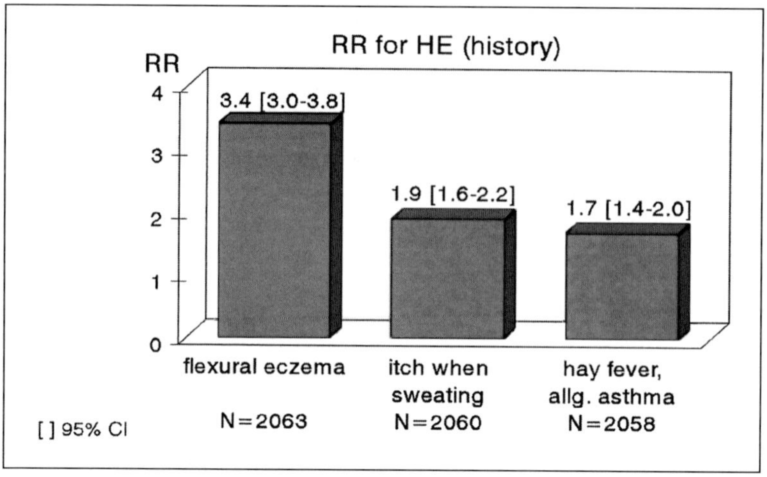

Fig. 5. Risk factors for HE (self-assessment). RR for HE (history).

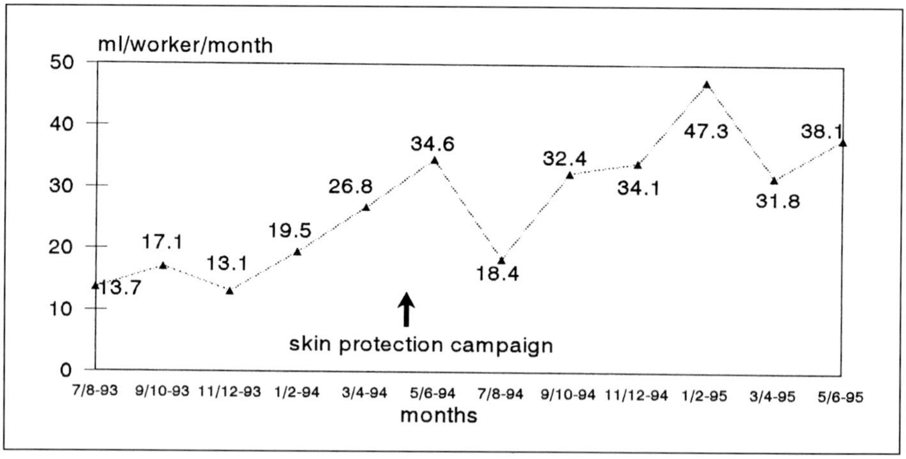

Fig. 6. Distribution of barrier creams. Motor and chassis parts manufacturing.

30.9% without a history of HE used the free available barrier creams twice a day or more (once a day or more: 72.0%/56.5%). Experience of HE was again the most important factor for the frequent use of barrier creams, but on the other hand 23.2% of the workers with a history of HE neither used barrier creams at the workplace nor at home.

For HE prevention it was therefore necessary to enforce the use of barrier creams especially in high-risk groups. Again supported by specially informed and trained team leaders as disseminators, the results of the campaign and the possibilities of HE prevention at the workplace were discussed at the team meetings. To analyze the success of this procedure and to give some basic information to the management, the amount of distributed barrier creams was evaluated regularly. After the skin protection campaign and the following team meetings in autumn 1994, the use of barrier creams could be elevated to a significantly higher level than before (fig. 6).

Conclusions

Predisposing factors and some domestic risk factors are important confounders of work-related ICD.

As skin protection measures are not sufficient even in high-risk groups for HE, the intervals of special periodical medical examinations must be adjusted for risk groups and degree of exposure to irritants.

Identification of high-risk groups for HE also can be evaluated by self-assessment.

The structure production teams can be used successfully to enforce the prevention of HE and ICD.

From the point of view of occupational medicine today and because of new knowledge and practical experience at the workplace some promising tools for the prevention of ICD have been developed. If these tools are used consequently the prevention of ICD may become one of the most exciting fields in occupational and preventive medicine.

Acknowledgments

The prospective cohort study is financially supported by grants from the German research minister (BMFT, Förderkennzeichen 01HK919/5 and 01HK899/3). The extensive study would not have been possible without the help of the observers from the Department of Dermatology of the University of Erlangen-Nuremberg and the Departments of Occupational Medicine of AUDI AG in Ingolstadt and Neckarsulm.

References

1 Funke U, Diepgen TL, Fartasch M: Identification of high-risk groups for irritant contact dermatitis by occupational physicians, in Elsner P, Maibach HI (eds): Irritant Dermatitis: New Clinical and Experimental Aspects. Curr Probl Dermatol. Basel, Karger, 1995, vol 23, pp 64–72.

2 Diepgen TL, Fartasch M, Hornstein OP: Evaluation and relevance of atopic basic and minor features in patients with atopic dermatitis and in the general population. Acta Derm Venerol 1989; (suppl 144):50–54.

3 Nilsson E, Mikaelsson B, Andersson S: Atopy, occupation and domestic work as risk factors for hand eczema in hospital workers. Contact Dermatitis 1985;13:216–223.

4 Funke U: Risikogruppenbezogene Prävention von Hautkrankheiten im Betrieb. Arbeitsmed Sozialmed Umweltmed 1995;30:257–264.

5 Kristensen O: A prospective study of the development of hand eczema in an automobile manufacturing industry. Contact Dermatitis 1992;26:341–345.

Dr. med. U. Funke, Gesundheitswesen AUDI AG, Postfach 10 02 20,
D–85045 Ingolstadt (Germany)

Elsner P, Lachapelle JM, Wahlberg JE, Maibach HI (eds): Prevention of
Contact Dermatitis. Curr Probl Dermatol. Basel, Karger, 1996, vol 25, pp 133–144

Risk Assessment and Exposure Control in an Occupational Setting

C.L. Packham

EnviroDerm Services, North Littleton, Evesham, UK

Risk assessment and exposure control are primary measures in the prevention of occupational dermatitis. Yet despite its significance, little technology exists to assist those responsible for monitoring and assessing skin exposure in the workplace. There are also no data readily available on the significance of a given level of exposure.

A structured approach, as described, assists in identifying the many complex ways in which exposure can occur and provides consistency in assessing relative significance.

Rules for controlling exposure commence with measures to make the workplace intrinsically safe for the skin. Measures such as provision of personal protective equipment and personal hygiene, whilst useful, are subsidiary to engineering control. Education and training, for both management and workforce, are key constituents of any effective programme to prevent occupational dermatitis.

Objectives

The main objective is to ensure that no-one's health is adversely affected as a result of contact between the skin and substances used in the workplace.

Subsidiary objectives might be to: (1) Identify all substances in the workplace and ascertain their potential to cause damage to health through contact with the skin. (2) Establish the level of exposure which is occurring – or might occur – and assess the affect on health which this might have. (3) Introduce measures to prevent such exposure occurring, or, where this is not possible, to limit it so that damage to health is avoided.

Risk Assessment

Risk vs. Hazard

We need to be clear on what is meant by the terms 'risk' and 'hazard'. The hazard presented by a substance is its intrinsic property to cause damage. The risk is the probability that in the circumstances actual damage to health will occur.

As an example, nitric acid is certainly hazardous. However, if it is only used in very small amounts in a closed system such that contact with employees is virtually excluded, then the risk will be extremely small.

The relationship between hazard and risk can be summarised as:

Risk = Hazard × Exposure.

Multiplicity of Risks

In any workplace different tasks will produce different risks. Each of these will require assessment. A risk assessment for that workplace will therefore be concerned with establishing the level of each risk and creating a priority list. This will enable risks to be dealt with in order of descending severity.

Assessment and Subjectivity

Any assessment is, by definition, subjective. If risks are to be ranked according to severity it is important that a consistent approach is adopted. Experience suggests that a structured approach, similar to that shown in figure 1, will help to ensure that no risk is given an unduly high priority.

Policy and Planning

Before assessment commences it is important to ensure that objectives have been clearly stated, agreed with management and communicated to all those concerned. Those responsible for conducting the assessment should ensure that they have the necessary training, equipment and knowledge of the workplace. They should also insist on having the required time and authority. These are important. To conduct a comprehensive risk assessment will take considerable time. Unless the assessor has the appropriate authority he or she may not be able to obtain the full co-operation of line management and workforce or access to adequate sources of information.

Consultation

Since risk assessment is concerned with what actually happens in the workplace it is logical to engage the support of those in the workplace on a daily basis. In practice, only the workforce themselves will know exactly what happens during the working day. Since many activities will occur only infre-

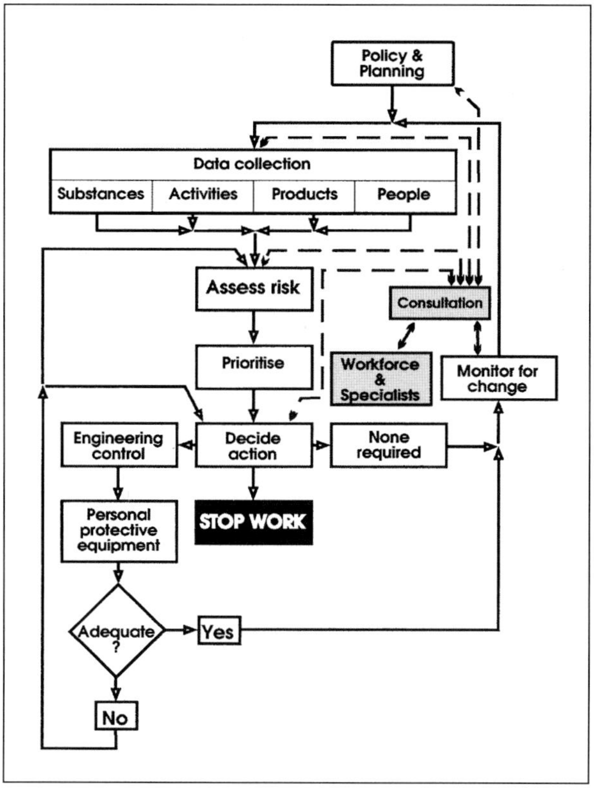

Fig. 1. Risk assessment.

quently, it may not be possible for the assessor to be present for each and every one. Thus, he or she will have to rely upon the information obtained from those actually carrying out the task.

This suggests that the workforce should be involved in the risk assessment from the outset. An additional benefit of this is that, by virtue of their involvement, they will feel a part ownership of the results. This makes it more probable that control measures introduced to rectify unsatisfactory situations will be adhered to.

Data Collection

Once the assessor, or assessment team, is ready to start, the first task will be to collect as much data as possible about the workplace and the activities that are carried out therein (fig. 2). We can divide this into four main categories: (1) substances; (2) activities; (3) products; (4) people.

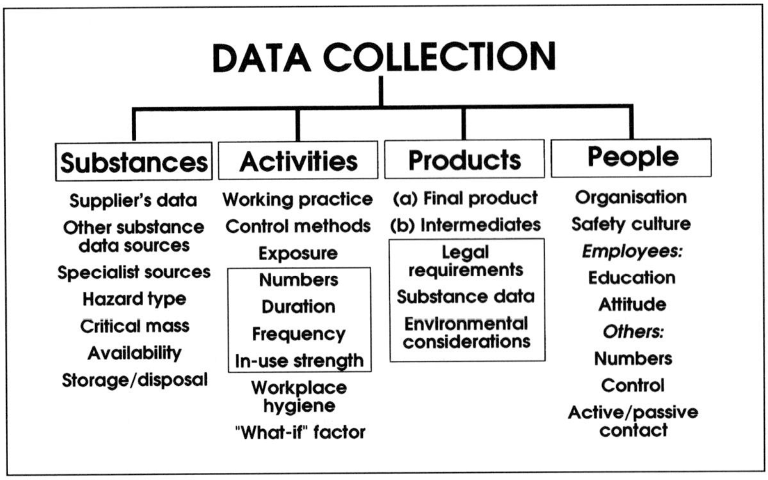

Fig. 2. Data collection.

'Substances' includes all those items brought into the workplace from outside, even if at first glance they may appear harmless. 'Activities' covers what actually happens within the establishment – or as a result of its operations. By 'products' we mean those items that the workplace produces, either as a finished product for sale or as an intermediate for subsequent processing within the workplace. 'People' falls into two categories, those employed and those who, whilst not employed, might be present in the workplace or be affected by its operations.

Substances. Start by making a list of all substances to be found in the workplace. No substance should be excluded at this stage on the basis that it is not hazardous. We now need to obtain data on the substance so that the hazards it represents can be identified.

Usually, the initial information is that provided by the supplier. This should be treated with caution. Errors and omissions are still commonplace. Do not rely upon the supplier's assurances that the substance is not hazardous. A list of ingredients is essential as it enables a check to be made on the validity of any such assurances.

This is not to suggest that the supplier is deliberately misleading his customers – although unfortunately this does still sometimes occur. We have to remember that the supplier is usually an expert in his particular field and not an expert in the complex field of occupational dermatology.

We may need then to refer to *specialist sources* such as a substance hazard database or the local skin clinic.

The *type of hazard* represented by the substance must be identified. It may be an irritant, a sensitizer or toxic. Of course, it may be more than one of these!

The next question is simply: 'How much is present?' If this is less than is needed to cause a problem (the *critical mass*) then the substance can probably be ignored.

The form in which the substance is present is also important. This is particularly true for sensitizers. Unless the substance is in a form in which it can penetrate the skin, i.e. 'available', then the risk of damage to health will probably be relatively small.

Many nickel-sensitive people can safely handle stainless steel, despite its high nickel content. This is because the nickel is so tightly bound into the steel that none is 'available' to penetrate the skin and trigger the allergic response.

Working Practice. As already stated, in most workplaces only the workforce themselves will actually know what happens. However, it is unwise to rely solely upon their description of the way a task is carried out. Even if they are genuinely attempting to describe the operation, experience suggests that what they will describe is what they think they do! Observation may reveal differences between this and the actual execution of the task. Equally, they may not be able to detect or identify potential sources of exposure.

Thus only observation over a period of time will reveal the true level of exposure. Since many tasks, such as machine setting, cleaning and maintenance, will only occur at infrequent intervals, it may be necessary to visit the same site within the workplace on several occasions. This may involve visits during a night shift or at week-ends. This is why adequate time must be allowed for a risk assessment.

Questions such as: 'Are there defined ways of doing the task?', i.e. is there a standard *working practice*, need to be addressed. Are control measures in place, e.g. splash guards, local exhaust ventilation? Are they working? How are they maintained? Are they fail-safe?

Can we identify any *exposure*? Some of the ways in which exposure can occur are identified in table 1.

The *number* of people exposed and the *duration* and *frequency* of the exposure should be noted.

Where substances are diluted for use, the technique for dilution should be ascertained. In many cases, such as with water-mixed metalworking fluids, regular checks on the condition of the liquid will be required. This will identify any change in mixture strength, bacterial contamination, etc.

The overall condition of the workplace (*workplace hygiene*) should be noted. Are machines and floors cleaned regularly or is debris and work in

Table 1. Routes of skin contact

Gas		
Airborne	–	direct
Airborne	–	indirect, e.g. absorption in substances handled, such as clothing, filters in masks
	–	condensation to liquid
Liquid		
Direct	–	through immersion
	–	as spray
	–	as condensation on cold surfaces
Indirect	–	contamination of clothing
	–	absorption of liquid into substances
Permeation	–	through gloves or other types of personal protective equipment
Solid		
Direct	–	as solid if sufficient free ions available
	–	as dust from mechanical action
	–	as fume or smoke particle from combustion (e.g. welding)
Indirect	–	as contamination in clothing
	–	as contamination in liquids (e.g. metals in metalworking fluids)

progress allowed to accumulate? This will provide a good indication of the care which is given to adherence to safe methods of work.

Finally, the *'what-if'* factor must be considered. All may appear in order now, but if, for example, two incompatible chemicals are stored in adjacent bays, what is the possibility of confusion and could an accident whereby they became mixed cause a potential hazard?

Products. Finished products will almost certainly have their own substance data sheet, if only because this is required by the customer. Intermediates are another question! Within the workplace two substances may be mixed, for subsequent use within the process. It is not uncommon to find data available for each substance (provided by the supplier), but none for the mixture. Yet the mixture may have very different properties from the original substances.

People. Questions should be asked about the way in which health and safety is organised within the workplace. Is there a general awareness among all that health and safety are everyone's concern? Or is this seen as the responsibility of the health and safety department or manager? The latter will almost certainly result in an upgrading of most of the risks found!

Do not overlook those who might have to visit the workplace from time to time, such as outside engineering consultants, service engineers, etc. What

Table 2. Rating of probability

Amost impossible	0
Exceptional, short term	1
Exceptional, extended	2
Improbable, short term	3
Improbable, extended	4
Probable, short term	5
Probable, extended	6
Highly probable, short term	7
Highly probable, extended	8
Common, frequent, short term	9
Common, frequent, extended	10

provisions does the organisation have to ensure that these people are not allowed to place themselves at risk, either deliberately or through ignorance of the hazards within the workplace?

Assess Risk. By comparison with the techniques and equipment available for monitoring and measuring respiratory exposure there is little to help the health and safety professional concerned with assessing the extent and significance of exposure of the skin to chemicals.

Those techniques which are available generally fall into two main categories. Some are relatively accurate but highly complex and really only suited for sophisticated, laboratory-based, research projects. Others, such as skin wipes, may be simpler to use but give only a basic indication of whether exposure is present or not. They will not indicate the level of exposure.

Thus, assessing skin exposure in the workplace will depend on keen observation, experience and judgement by the assessor based on his knowledge of the process and the substances in use. Past history, such as reports of problems with similar processes elsewhere, can be of significant help, but may be difficult, or time consuming, to obtain.

Since in any normal workplace there will be a multiplicity of risks of varying degrees of severity, risk assessment is really about ordering these by severity so that the most serious risks are dealt with first. We therefore need a simple, structured approach to rank risks to the skin in order of severity. Since, by definition, risk assessment will be subjective, it is important that the system is so structured to ensure consistency when assessing individual risks.

Prioritise. One method of encouraging this is to divide the assessment into two components, probability and effect. These can then be rated using the scales shown in tables 2 and 3. The nomogramme in figure 3 will then

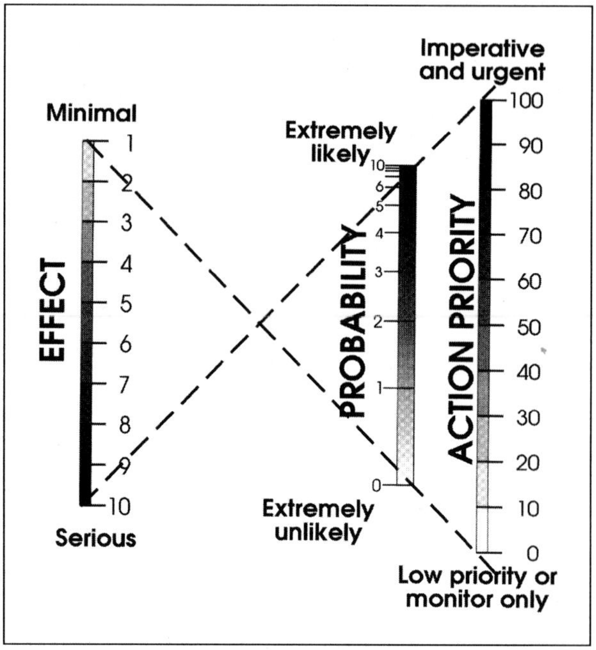

Fig. 3. Chart for rating risk severity.

Table 3. Rating of effect

Fatal Irreversible, total or severe	10
Irrreversible, moderate Reversible, long term, total or severe	9
Reversible, long term, moderate Reversible, medium term, severe	8
Irreversible, slight Reversible, medium term, moderate Reversible, short term, severe Reversible, long term, slight	7
Reversible, medium term, slight Reversible, short term, moderate	5
Reversible, short term, slight	2
Virtually none – or insignificant	1

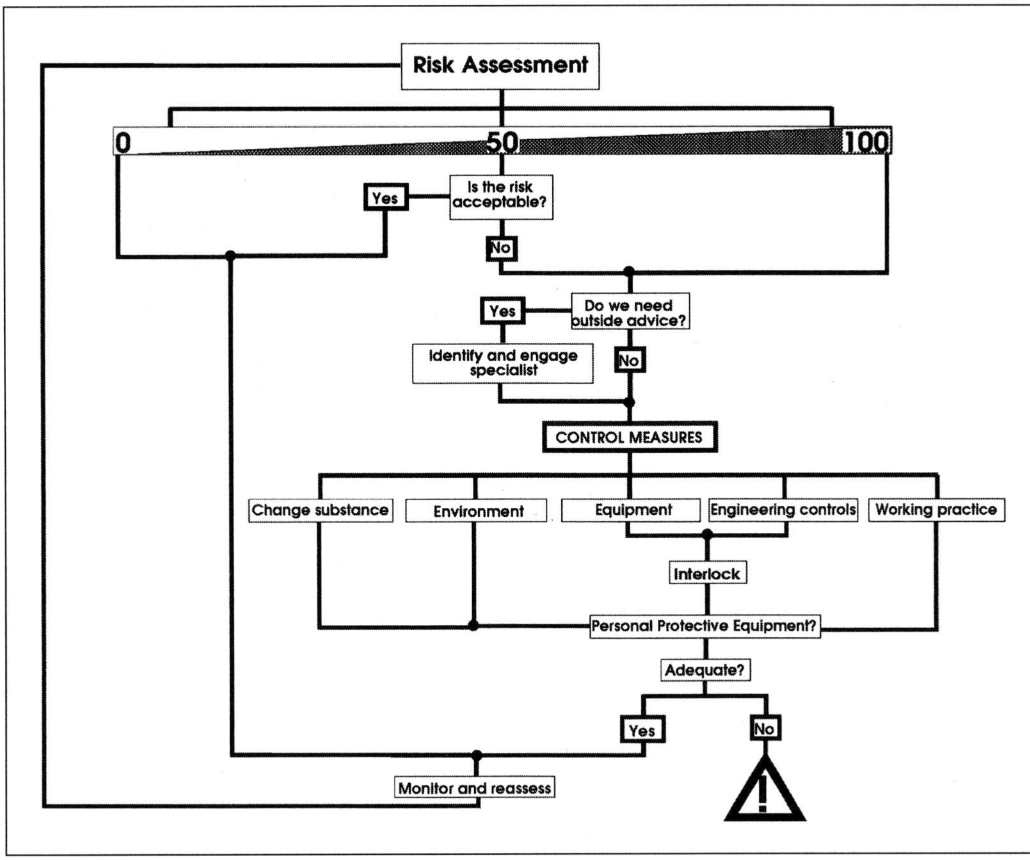

Fig. 4. Identification, rating and control of risk.

enable a relative risk value to be determined. The risk can then be allocated its correct place within the priority list.

Decide Action. Risk assessment is not an end in itself. It is only a means to identify and prioritise risks for the purposes of introducing and maintaining adequate control so that damage to health does not occur. Therefore, having assessed our risks, and commencing with the ones with the highest rating, we need to decide upon the action to take to achieve such control.

It is good practice, once control measures have been introduced, to re-assess the risk and allocate it a new rating. This ensures both that we have an indication of the effectiveness of our control measures and that we develop a 'rolling effect' in our list of risks so that we are continuously striving to create a workplace with minimum overall risk to health.

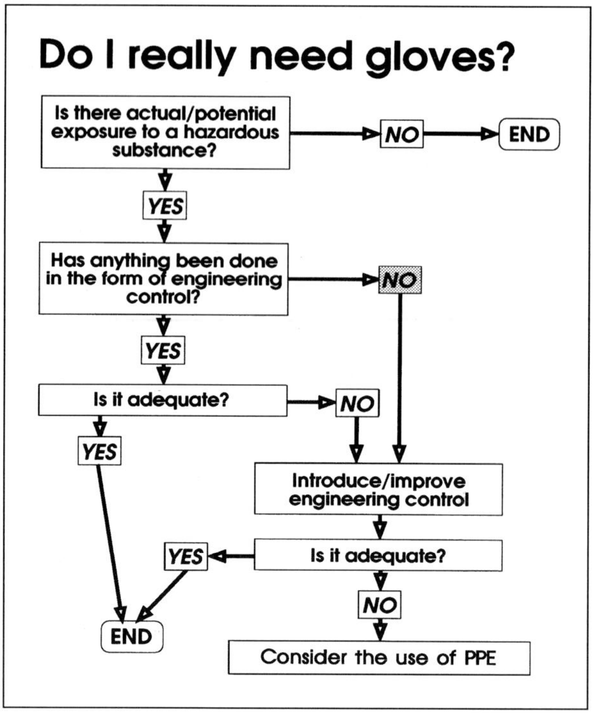

Fig. 5. Glove selection. Do I really need gloves?

Table 4. Exposure control strategy

Workplace and machinery design
Workplace culture
Education and training (management – workforce – outworkers)
Substances
Engineering controls
Working practice
Personal protection
Personal hygiene
Feedback and monitoring (health surveillance)
Problem identification and investigation

Table 5. Glove selection

What factors does my glove system need to take into account?	
1	Does the use of gloves introduce a potential new hazard?
2	Is there potential for confusion?
3	Do I need to provide training?
4	What do I need to do about control and maintenance?
5	What are the consequences of failure?
6	Have I made adequate provision for 'feedback' so if there is a problem with gloves it can be addressed?
7	What are the cost implications?

Exposure Control

As figure 4 shows, there are several ways in which exposure control can be achieved. Table 4 indicates a possible sequence of methods. These are shown in descending order of preference.

Engineering Control

The basic rulses for any control strategy should be: (1) control the process not the person, and (2) make the system fail-safe (so far as this is possible).

Controlling the process eliminates the uncertainty introduced by human unpredictability. It also makes it easier to develop systems which are fail-safe. Splash guards, for example, can be interlocked with the machine so that the latter will only operate with the guards in place. Sensors can be fitted to local exhaust ventilation systems so that if these are not functioning adequately the process is shut down, or at least a warning is given.

Working Practice

By contrast, relying on the worker, however skilled and well motivated, to carry out a task correctly, possibly many times during a day, can seldom be fail-safe. Even protective gloves, however carefully selected, will expose the worker if damaged or used incorrectly.

Personal Protective Equipment

Selection and use of personal protective equipment is not a simple task. Many factors will influence whether this will work as intended or required. Figure 5 shows the initial considerations, i.e. whether personal protective equipment is actually required.

Table 5 shows some of the considerations. We must ensure that, when recommending personal protective equipment, it not only works but does not introduce new hazards. These could include accidents caused by a loss of dexterity or agility, allergic reactions to the material from which the equipment is made and effects on the wearer, such as heat stress.

Conclusions

Assessing risks to the skin in the workplace is not a simple task. Until such time as simple, effective monitoring and measuring techniques become available, much will depend upon the knowledge and experience of the assessor. Almost invariably such an assessment will take considerably more time than might, at first, appear necessary.

Obtaining adequate information on the substances present in the workplace is also not easy. We lack a simple, comprehensive and up-to-date database on hazards presented by substances to the skin.

However, by following basic rules there is no doubt that risk assessment and exposure control can play a major role in reducing the unacceptably high incidence of occupational skin disease.

C.L. Packham, EnviroDerm Services, 2 Amery Lodge Farm, North Littleton, Evesham WR11 5QN (UK)

Elsner P, Lachapelle JM, Wahlberg JE, Maibach HI (eds): Prevention of Contact Dermatitis. Curr Probl Dermatol. Basel, Karger, 1996, vol 25, pp 145–153

Secondary Prevention: Detection of the Allergen

Ann-Therese Karlberg, Elisabeth Gäfvert

Department of Occupational Dermatology, National Institute for Working Life, Solna, Sweden

For prevention and treatment of allergic contact dermatitis, the major steps to be taken are to identify, detect and avoid the offending agent. Preferably, the agent should be eliminated from the products of interest or its allergenic capacity should be diminished by chemical means. Methods need to be developed to identify allergens. For some well-known allergens there exist spot tests which are described in textbooks [1], but also more sophisticated analytical methods. Many technical products contain several components and also contaminants that could sensitize the patient. In complex natural materials such as balsam of Peru and colophony, the patients could become sensitized to different allergens. To identify the actual sensitizer is often impossible, but selected markers can be detected that indicate the presence of allergenic components (e.g. abietic acid as a marker for the presence of allergenic colophony components).

Patch testing is used to detect contact allergy to a specific substance. A standard series of the most common contact allergens in society is used as a first screening. When a patient reacts to a patch test in this series it is important to know and inform of the prevalence of the allergen in the environment. General information about each allergen in the standard series and the products in which the allergen may be present is often compilated in info sheets and can be handed over to the patient with a brief discussion. However, if the patient needs exact knowledge of what products in his own environment are causing the dermatitis it is necessary to perform a more thorough investigation. This includes chemical analysis to detect the allergen in the products and patch testing with these products.

Patch testing with the patient's own products can often be rather complicated. Components with irritating potential interfere with the positive allergic patch test result and the product may need to be diluted to avoid irritation.

However, a false-negative reaction can be the result when the product is diluted too much. If possible, the ingredients of a product suspected to give allergic contact dermatitis should be tested separately. Requests of ingredients are time consuming and not all producers are willing to submit the information.

Analytical Methods Used at the Clinic

For some allergens there exist simple spot tests that could be used at the clinic and by the patients themselves. The most common is the dimethylglyoxime test for *nickel*. Dimethylglyoxime reacts with nickel ions in the presence of ammonia giving a salt with a bright red color. The sensitivity of the test can be enhanced by pretreatment of the object's surface with a solution of synthetic sweat and heat. The test has been proposed as a screening test for nickel release from jewelry and alloys by CEN/TC 283 (European Committee for Standardization).

Another well-known method is the detection of *formaldehyde* using chromotropic acid. A sample of the product, e.g. shampoo, cutting fluid or a skin care product, is put in a glass test tube and the chromotropic acid in sulfuric acid is put into another test tube. Both test tubes are placed in a closed glass stoppered jar and kept in the dark. The formaldehyde present will evaporate from the product and react with the chromotropic acid in the other test tube producing a violet-colored derivative. By comparing the intensity of the color with the colors from a series of standard solutions of formaldehyde it is possible to make a semiquantitative determination. A higher content of formaldehyde gives a more intense violet color. The presence of other low-molecular-weight aldehydes and ketones will interfere in the analysis since they will also react with chromotropic acid giving derivatives of different colors.

Epoxy oligomers of bisphenol A type could be detected using a simple thin-layer chromatography (TLC) method [2]. The oligomers are separated on the TLC plate showing a band of bright red spots each spot representing oligomers with the same mean molecular weight. A resin or a product suspected to contain an epoxy resin obtained from a patient is compared with a standard solution of the oligomers.

Chemical Analysis Performed in the Laboratory

A thorough investigative analytical work requires access to more sophisticated equipment. Two analytical methods of importance are high-performance liquid chromatography (HPLC) and gas chromatography (GC). *Formaldehyde* and other aldehydes can be detemined quantitatively using HPLC. Aliphatic aldhydes are reacted with 2,4-dinitrophenylhydrazine to get detectable UV absorption [3]. Using this method we have determined formaldehyde in non-ionic tensides. The knowledge that formaldehyde could be present in tensides is important, because it shows an allergenic contribution to the contact dermatitis caused by wetwork in formaldehyde-sensitive subjects and could thus aggravate the dermatitis. The official EEC method for detection of formaldehyde is by reaction with acetylacetone yielding the yellow derivative lutidine (2,6-dimethyl-3,5-diacetyldihydro-pyridine) [4]. However, with the described methods it is not possible to determine the amount of free formaldehyde in products containing *formaldehyde donors* as preservatives, since the methods will determine all formaldehyde that could be released from the donors. The official EEC method to detect free formaldehyde in the presence of formaldehyde donors is a complicated HPLC method including postcolumn derivatisation and extensive temperature control of the system [5]. The donor and free formaldehyde are separated on a column and the eluting formaldehyde is reacted with acetylacetone. At our laboratory we are at present developing a simple method to determine free formaldehyde directly in the presence of the donor. The amount of formaldehyde released from formaldehyde donors such as diazolidinyl urea (Germall II) and imidazolidinyl urea (Germall 115) is dependent on the pH value of the product; the higher the pH value, the higher the content of free formaldehyde. In addition to the allergenic activity of the donor itself; it is therefore important to be aware that formaldehyde could contribute to the allergenic effect in products with neutral or alkaline pH values. Patch testing with formaldehyde is often rather difficult to reproduce and false-negative results could be obtained in patients with a true allergy. Besides patch testing with a serial dilution of formaldehyde it is advisable to perform chemical analyses of the suspected products using either simple semiquantitative methods or HPLC to determine the exposure in the patients' environment.

Colophony could be present in cosmetics such as mascara, rouge and lipstick to make the products stick to the skin. Using HPLC, colophony components in mascaras of different brands have been detected (fig. 1) [6, 7]. The mascaras gave positive patch test reactions in colophony-sensitive subjects. The brands containing colophony could be found among the more exclusive ones and the statements of the producers are not always in accordance with reality. Some of the products were stated to be hypoallergenic and allergy tested. Colophony components were detected in a mascara used by a patient with eyelid dermatitis who had become sensitized to colophony in her work with colophony containing soldering fluxes. She changed to an office-type work but her dermatitis did not heal. The patient then blamed her visual

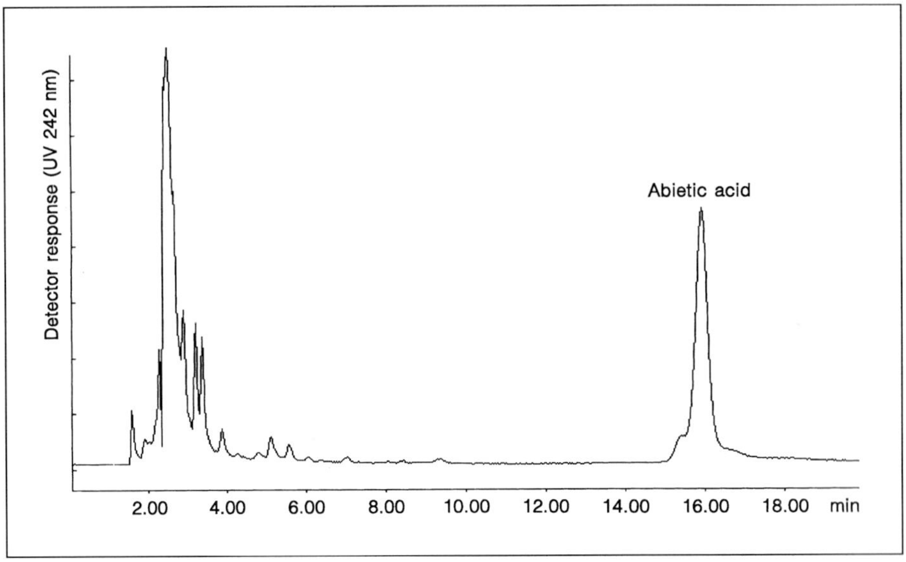

Fig. 1. HPLC analysis of a mascara according to the method described by Ehrin and Karlberg [6]. Abietic acid was observed in the methanol extract at retention time 16 min.

display unit. Her dermatitis healed when she stopped using her mascara. Cases of eyelid dermatitis were reported from an office in Sweden and suspected to be part of a so-called 'sick building syndrome'. One of the subjects was allergic to colophony. Abietic acid, the main component in colophony was detected in the floor polish that was crackled and could be seen as a white powder on the office floor.

Identification of New Allergens in Complex Materials

In complex materials different compounds could be responsible for the allergenic effect. Advanced methods for isolation and structure elucidation must be used in the work to detect and identify the allergens. It is often necessary to synthesize larger amounts of the identified compound to be able to perform appropriate experimental sensitization studies. This is no longer a routine work that should be performed for the investigation of individual patients, but is demanded in more extensive research work.

Colophony has a complex composition consisting mainly of resin acids. The allergenic components were isolated using preparative HPLC and structure elucidation was performed with mass spectrometry (MS) and nuclear magnetic

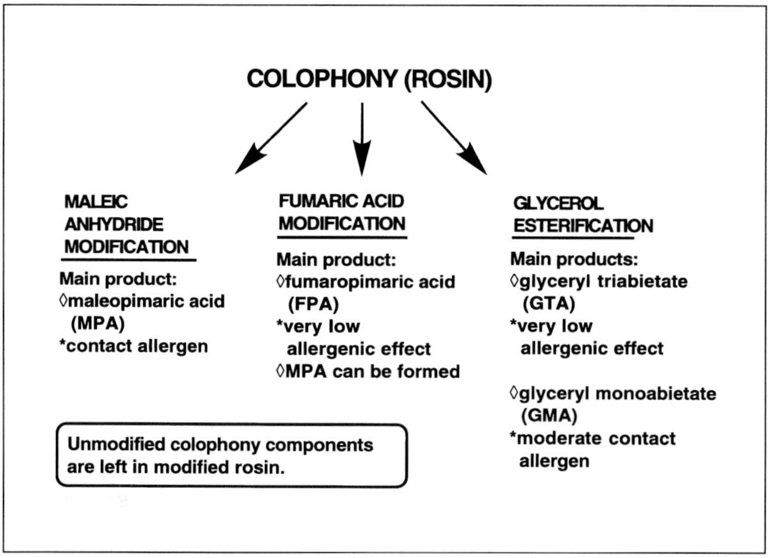

Fig. 2. Chemical modification of colophony creates new contact allergens not cross-reacting with the allergens in the unmodified colophony.

resonance (NMR). The sensitizing capacity of the compounds was determined in experimental studies in guinea pigs. The compounds were also tested in patients with known contact allergy to colophony [8–10]. Up to 70% of the patients reacted to single allergens, but for screening purposes the colophony as such still detects more cases of contact allergy [11]. However, most colophony is chemically modified to obtain suitable technical properties. New allergens were detected in the modified products using the same technique that was used for detection and identification of the allergens in unmodified colophony (fig. 2). The new allergens are not cross-reacting with the allergens in unmodified colophony [12]. Screening with the allergens identified in modified colophony detects cases of contact allergy that are not revealed when testing only with unmodified colophony.

HPLC was the method of choice when components with sensitizing capacity were detected in *phenol formaldehyde resins* and in products containing these resins [13]. The sensitizers were detected in decorative laminate, casting sand, mineral wool and masonite using reversed-phase HPLC. Allergenic components were identified as isomers of methylol phenols and dihydroxy diphenylmethanes using MS and NMR. The identified components were tested in patients with contact allergy to phenol formaldehyde resin and with an occupational exposure to this type of resins. Over 60% of the patients reacted to

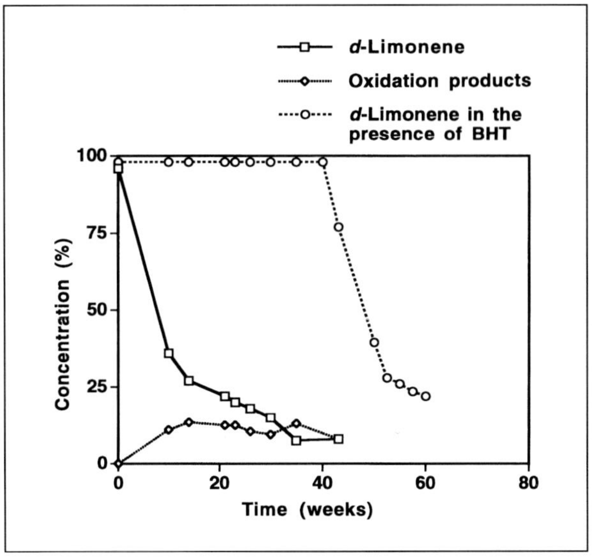

Fig. 3. Air oxidation of *d*-limonene. Degradation of *d*-limonene and formation of oxidation products.

at least one of the tested components. Different components evoked reactions in different individuals [14]. This knowledge together with the observation that the amount and identity of the sensitizers varied from one phenol formaldehyde resin to another showed that using only one type of resin for patch testing will not reveal all cases of this contact allergy.

Identification of the True Allergen

It might not be the substance itself that is the offending allergen. Impurities or oxidation products formed by air exposure could be the true causes of the allergy. *d*-Limonene (orange peel oil) has long been used in low concentrations as a perfume in many products such as shampoos and cleaning agents. In recent years, it has been heavily advertised as an environmentally friendly substituent for other organic solvents and defatting agents in the industry. The concentrations of *d*-limonene in such products could vary between 20 and 100%. Thus, the exposure will be quite different compared to the earlier usage. In our research on the allergenicity of *d*-limonene we have seen that *d*-limonene is not stable when handled. In a simple model to mimic the handling in the industry, we found that *d*-limonene is easily oxidized at air

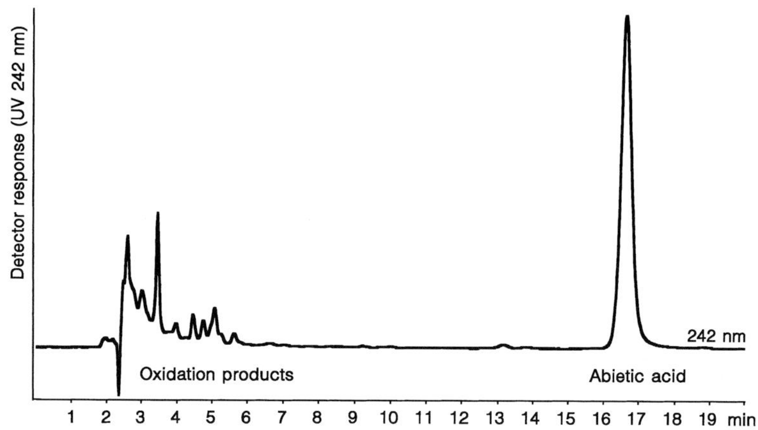

Fig. 4. HPLC analysis of abietic acid of commercial quality. The purity of abietic acid was 40% according to the analysis.

exposure (fig. 3). The oxidation products formed were found to be allergenic while *d*-limonene itself showed a very low sensitizing capacity [15, 16]. Patch testing with oxidized *d*-limonene reveals new cases of contact allergy not identified with the standard allergens. To prevent from relapsing dermatitis the patient then has to avoid products containing *d*-limonene. In this case the nose is an excellent detector, since the smell of lemon is very easily distinguished.

Abietic acid, the main component in colophony, is another example of a compound which itself is a very weak sensitizer, but on contact with air forms several oxidation products with high sensitizing capacity [8]. Abietic acid is very easily oxidized in contact with air and a newly purified sample will immediately start to degrade. The abietic acid used for patch testing is not pure but contains considerable amounts of oxidation products. An HPLC analysis of a commercially available test substance showed that only 40% of the sample was unoxidized abietic acid (fig. 4).

When the allergenicity of a product is mainly due to its oxidation products it is important to diminish the oxidation. Such a product should therefore be stored dark and cold, when not used. Furthermore, it should not be used for a long time without analyzing the purity. One way to diminish the allergenic activity of compounds and products that easily form allergenic oxidation products is to add antioxidants. Adding butylated hydroxytoluene (BHT) to *d*-limonene prevents the formation of oxidation products and thus the allergenicity is kept at a low level (fig. 3) [17]. BHT itself is a weak allergen [18].

Conclusion

The detection and identification of the offending allergen in the products in the patient's environment both at home and at work is an important part of the preventive work dealing with allergic contact dermatitis. The methods could be simple spot tests or documented analytical methods including HPLC and GC when the allergen is well known. For identification of new allergens sophisticated methods for isolation and structure elucidation have to be performed. Identification of the true allergens is important not only for the single patient but also in the work to prevent products with allergenic properties to enter the market.

References

1 Wall LM: Spot tests and chemical analyses for allergen evaluation; in Rycroft RJG, Menné T, Frosch PJ (eds): Testbook of Contact Dermatitis, ed 2. Berlin, Springer, 1995, pp 277–285.

2 Fregert S, Trulson L: Simple methods for demonstrating of epoxy resin of bisphenol A type. Contact Dermatitis 1978;4:69–72.

3 Selim S: Separation and quantitative determination of traces of carbonyl compounds as their 2,4-dinitrophenylhydrazones by high-pressure liquid chromatography. J Chromatogr 1977;136:271–277.

4 Commission Directive 90/207/EEC amending the Second Directive 82/434/EEC on the approximation of the laws of the Member State relating to methods of analysis necessary for checking the composition of cosmetic products. Official J Eur Commun 1990;No L 108:92–101.

5 Engelhardt H, Klinker R: Determination of free formaldehyde in the presence of donators in cosmetics by HPLC and post-column derivation. Chromatographia 1985;20:559–565.

6 Ehrin E, Karlberg A-T: Detection of rosin (colophony) components in technical products using an HPLC technique. Contact Dermatitis 1990;23:359–366.

7 Karlberg A-T, Lidén C, Ehrin E: Colophony in mascara as a cause of eye-lid dermatitis. Acta Derm Venereol 1991;71:445–447.

8 Karlberg A-T: Contact allergy to colophony: Chemical identifications of allergens, sensitization experiments and clinical experiences. Acta Derm Venereol 1988;(suppl 139):1–43.

9 Gäfvert E, Nilsson U, Karlberg A-T, Magnusson K, Nilsson JLG: Rosin allergy: Identification of a dehydroabietic acid peroxide with allergenic properties. Arch Dermatol Res 1992;284:409–413.

10 Gäfvert E, Shao LP, Karlberg A-T, Nilsson U, Nilsson JLG: Contact allergy to resin acid hydroperoxides: Hapten binding via free radicals and epoxides. Chem Res Toxicol 1994;7:260–266.

11 Karlberg A-T, Gäfvert E: Isolated rosin (colophony) allergens as screening substances for contact allergy. Contact Dermatitis, in press.

12 Gäfvert E: Allergenic components in modified and unmodified rosin: Chemical characterization and studies of allergenic activity. Acta Derm Venereol 1994;(suppl 184):1–36.

13 Bruze M, Persson L, Trulson L, Zimerson E: Demonstration of contact sensitizers in resins and products based on phenol-formaldehyde. Contact Dermatitis 1986;14:146–154.

14 Bruze M, Contact sensitizers in resins based on phenol and formaldehyde. Thesis Lund 1985. Acta Derm Venereol 1986;(suppl 119):1–36.
15 Karlberg A-T, Magnusson K, Nilsson U: Air oxidation of *d*-limonene – the citrus solvent – creates potent allergens. Contact Dermatitis 1992;26:332–340.
16 Karlberg A-T, Shao LP, Nilsson U, Gäfvert E, Nilsson JLG: Hydroperoxides in oxidized *d*-limonene identified as potent contact allergens. Arch Dermatol Res 1994;286:97–103.
17 Karlberg A-T, Magnusson K, Nilsson U: Influence of an antioxidant on the formation of allergenic compounds during autoxidation of *d*-limonene. Ann Occup Hyg 1994;38:199–207.
18 Flyvholm M-A, Menné T: Sensitizing risk of butylated hydroxytoluene based on exposure and effect data. Contact Dermatitis 1990;23:341–345.

Dr. Ann-Therese Karlberg, Department of Occupational Dermatology,
National Institute for Working Life, S–171 84 Solna (Sweden)

Elsner P, Lachapelle JM, Wahlberg JE, Maibach HI (eds): Prevention of Contact Dermatitis. Curr Probl Dermatol. Basel, Karger, 1996, vol 25, pp 154–162

Prognosis of Contact Dermatitis following Secondary Preventive Measures

C.L. Goh

Institute of Dermatology, Singapore National Skin Centre, Singapore

Persistence of dermatitis after avoidance of primary contactants is well known. Prognosis in contact dermatitis refers to the outcome of dermatitis over time with and without intervention. Understanding the prognosis of contact dermatitis enables the dermatologists to forecast probable outcome of the dermatitis to patients. Information on the prognosis helps dermatologists to (a) implement risk management of patients who are exposed to potential irritants and allergens; and (b) plan preventive measures against contact dermatitis. It also helps the relevant authorities to prioritise implementation of preventive measures.

Long-term outcome of contact dermatitis, especially occupational contact dermatitis, has important medicolegal implications. It helps dermatologists and occupational physicians to determine medicolegal compensation.

Unfortunately, long-term follow-up studies on prognosis of contact dermatitis, especially prospective studies, are often difficult because of (a) difficulty in recalling patients for follow-up; (b) difficulty in getting patients to go for clinical assessment; (c) difficulty in finding control groups for comparison, and (d) lack of accurate clinical data recordings.

Most reports on the prognosis rely on retrospective studies, most are derived from case records from contact and occupational skin disease clinics. Such data are generally biased and tend to include a selected cohort of patients who tend to have persistent or severe contact dermatitis or those who are likely to seek compensation. Most of the available reports on prognosis of contact dermatitis are based on reports from occupational contact dermatitis rather than nonoccupational dermatitis because of the medicolegal implications involved with occupational contact dermatitis.

Table 1. Prognosis of contact dermatitis: summary of studies

Author	Cohort	Type of dermatitis	Follow-up years	Clearance %
Skog and Tottie [1]	68	ACD/ICD	4–31	24
Agrup [2]	501	ACD/ICD	0.5–2	10
Burrows [3]	113	ACD/ICD	10–13	20
Fregert [4]	555	ACD/ICD	2–3	20, 29
Coenraads [6]	105	all	3	33
Schubert et al. [7]	104	ACD	3	8
Pryce et al. [8]	100	oil	1–5	25
Chia and Goh [9]	31/81	ACD/ICD	1	77/70
Rosen and Freeman [10]	336	ACD/ICD	1–5	38/30
Nethercott and Holness [11]	96/105	ACD/ICD	2	71/55

ACD = Allergic contact dermatitis; ICD = irritant contact dermatitis.

This chapter reviews the prognosis of patients with contact dermatitis following secondary preventive measures. Contact dermatitis outcome following secondary preventive measures refers to those of patients who were confirmed to have contact dermatitis based on clinical findings and those who had received appropriate management and received counselling on avoidance of contactants and on preventive measures. Association of prognosis outcome with risk factors including atopy, job change, age, contactants (irritants and allergens), and occupation will be presented.

Epidemiology

Most earlier reports on the prognosis of contact dermatitis (especially occupational contact dermatitis) documented poor prognosis for total clearance of dermatitis [1–8]. However, recent reports have indicated that the prognosis is much better [9–11]. The reported prognosis on clearance of dermatitis in patients with contact dermatitis follow-up over different periods varies from 8 to 77% [1–11].

Table 1 shows prognosis on total clearance of contact dermatitis from different studies from different countries.

It can be seen that the prognosis reported in the earlier years were generally poorer than those reported in recent years. Reports between 1961 and 1989 documented the prognosis for total clearance ranging from 8 to 33%. Reports after 1990 documented a clearance rate of about 70%.

Burrows [3] in 1972 reported that 79% of patients who were followed up over 10–13 years still required treatment for their contact dermatitis.

In Singapore, total clearance of dermatitis after 1 year of follow-up of patients with occupational contact dermatitis was 72% with slightly better prognosis for patients with allergic contact dermatitis (77%) than irritant contact dermatitis (70%). However, the difference was not statistically significant [9].

In Sydney, Rosen and Freeman [10] reported total clearance of dermatitis in 38% of patients with allergic contact dermatitis and 30% for patients with irritant contact dermatitis over a 2- to 10-year follow-up period. However, if patients who reported improvement were included as a favorable prognosis, then the rates were 74 and 68%, respectively.

In the United States, Nethercott and Holness [11] reported clearance in 63% of patients with occupational contact dermatitis followed up over 4 years. When patients with mild eczema were included, the improvement rate was 81%. There were more workers with allergic contact dermatitis who reported that they were free of dermatitis than irritant contact dermatitis in the study.

It appears that prognosis from contact dermatitis has improved in recent years. This could be due to several factors including (a) earlier diagnosis; (b) better management, and (c) better health education on preventive measures.

It also appeared that patients with allergic contact dermatitis have slightly better prognosis than those with irritant contact dermatitis. One reason could be because of the availability of the patch test to identify the specific causative allergen. The patient can then be counselled on the avoidance of the specific causative allergen. On the contrary, the cause of irritant contact dermatitis is often vague, multifactorial and very often these patients suffer from an underlying endogenous dermatitis which tends to perpetuate their dermatitis.

Prognosis and Age

The age of onset of contact dermatitis does not appear to influence its prognosis. Burrows [3] reported no significant difference in the prognosis between affected patients of <40 years old and those >40 years old (dermatitis clearance rate was 15 vs. 16%, respectively) followed up over 10–13 years.

Similarly, Pryce et al. [8] in their report on prognosis of occupational dermatitis from soluble oil showed no difference in prognosis for patients who are <50 years old and those >49 years old.

Chia and Goh [9] reported a slight improvement in prognosis in the older patients (>39 years old) with a clearance rate of 85% compared with those in younger patients with a clearance rate of 65%. The difference was not statistically significant.

Nethercott and Holness [11] also did not find any difference in prognosis among patients with contact dermatitis among different age groups.

Prognosis and Sex

Most reports showed that there was no significant difference in the prognosis of patients with contact dermatitis between males and females. In Singapore, the prognosis of male patients with allergic contact dermatitis (clearance rate of 90%) was significantly better than females (clearance rate of 50%). There was no significant difference in the clearance rate of irritant contact dermatitis between male and female patients (73 and 69%, respectively) [9].

Similarly, Nethercott and Holness [11] reported no significance difference in the prognosis of males and females with occupational contact dermatitis followed up over 2 years (with clearance rates of 60% for males vs. 75% for females).

Prognosis in Irritant and Allergic Contact Dermatitis

Prognosis of irritant contact dermatitis appears to be slightly poorer than for allergic contact dermatitis. Some occupational irritants appear more likely to lead to chronicity than others. In Singapore, cutting fluids and solvent-induced irritant contact dermatitis is associated with poor prognosis with about 40% of workers having persistent dermatitis after 1 year of follow-up even when they stopped working with the irritants [9]. Irritant dermatitis and cement irritant contact dermatitis from acids/alkali and cement appeared to have good prognosis in Singapore where all patients had clearance of their dermatitis when they stopped exposure to the irritant [9]. Patients who continued being exposed to these irritants had an even higher rate of persistent dermatitis (38% for cutting fluids and 58% for solvents). All patients with irritant contact dermatitis from other irritants including acids/alkali and cement had good prognosis despite continued exposure to the irritants.

Unlike allergic contact dermatitis from cement, irritant contact dermatitis from cement is associated with a good prognosis. In Singapore, all construction workers with irritant contact dermatitis from cement had complete clearance of their dermatitis despite continuation of work. Similarly, in Denmark irritant contact dermatitis from cement cleared in 80% of workers despite continuing the same job [12].

In Sydney, 30% of patients with irritant contact dermatitis had total clearance of dermatitis (2–10 years follow-up). Again, allergic contact dermatitis had a slightly better prognosis with a clearance rate of 38% [10].

Similarly, Nethercott and Holness [11] in the United States also reported better prognosis in patients with allergic contact dermatitis (clearance rate after 4 years of follow-up was 70%) compared to patients with irritant contact dermatitis (with a clearance rate of 58%).

Chia and Goh [9] reported that the overall prognosis from occupational allergic contact dermatitis was good with 77% of their patients reporting total clearance of dermatitis. However, patients with metal allergy, e.g. nickel and cobalt, had a poor prognosis. 75% of patients with metal allergy had persistent dermatitis despite 'avoidance' of metals. Similarly, rubber chemical allergies appeared to be associated with poor prognosis with a chronicity rate of 50%. One reason for the chronicity in contact allergy to these allergens could be due to their ubiquity. Daily avoidance of these allergens is almost impossible. Prognosis from other allergens, e.g. epoxy resin allergy, was good.

In contrast to previous reports on chromate dermatitis, the prognosis of patients with chromate dermatitis in Singapore was reported to be good. All 5 patients with chromate allergy had clearance of dermatitis upon avoidance of chromate [9].

Cement dermatitis from chromate allergy from cement is often associated with very poor prognosis. Burrows [3] reported that only 8% of patients with cement dermatitis had clearance of dermatitis after 10–13 years follow-up. In Sydney, the prognosis from chromate allergy was reported to be the worst among allergies to other occupational allergens with clearance rates of only <20% (over 2–10 years' follow-up period). In the report of Rosen and Freeman [10], clearance from contact allergy to *p*-phenylenediamine gave the best prognosis with clearance rates of about 50%.

Similar poor prognosis from cement dermatitis was reported in Perth, Australia, where 89% of cement workers with chromate allergy had persistent dermatitis when followed up between 6 months and 9 years [13].

In Denmark, follow-up of patients with chromate allergy after the introduction of ferrous sulfate in Danish cement to reduce hexavalent chromate concentration in cement continued to show poor prognosis. Only 30% of workers who remained on the job had total clearance of their dermatitis [12]. It would appear that chromate dermatitis is associated with poor prognosis. Avoidance of chromates in cement does not appear to reduce chronicity. One reason for chronicity could be due to the ubiquitous nature of chromate in our environment.

Prognosis and Occupation

Among the occupational group, construction workers with contact dermatitis were consistently reported to have the worse prognosis [3, 4, 10, 12]. The clearance rates over 2–9 years' follow-up for construction workers in Sydney was <20% compared to clearance rates of 40% among medical workers and 35% among hairdressers and food handlers [10]. When improvements were considered a good prognosis, the improvement rates for construction workers remained lower at 40% compared to rates of about 80% for medical workers, hairdressers and food handlers [10].

Pryce et al. [8] reported that cutting fluid dermatitis among metalworkers tends to persist with overall clearance rates of about 20% during a 2-year follow-up.

Hairdressers with irritant contact dermatitis also appeared to have good prognosis when they change jobs. Matsunaga et al. [14] reported a 70% clearance rate for hairdressers who stopped working in their profession.

Prognosis and Job Change

Most patients with contact dermatitis who changed their jobs did so for reasons other than dermatitis [2, 5, 15]. There were conflicting reports indicating that job change affected prognosis. Most earlier reports indicated that job change is not associated with significant improvement in the prognosis of occupational contact dermatitis [2, 4, 5, 15–18]. However, there is a general tendency for improvement of dermatitis to occur among workers who changed their jobs. In most instances patients with occupational contact dermatitis continued to work despite their dermatitis. This stresses the importance for dermatologists to differentiate medical from social prognosis [19]. Many patients prefer to continue working despite their dermatitis.

Burrows [3] reported that only 20% of workers with dermatitis had stopped working when followed-up over 10–13 years of follow-up. Among these workers only 18% had clearance of their dermatitis.

Pryce et al. [8] reported persistence of dermatitis after 2 years of follow-up to be 88% for those who continued to be exposed to cutting fluid and 70% for those no longer exposed to cutting fluid.

Among hairdressers with occupational dermatitis, job change appears to confer good prognosis. Matsunaga et al. [14] from Japan reported clearance of dermatitis in 70% of beauticians who stopped work compared to 20% clearance rates in those who continued to work.

In Singapore, prognosis for patients with contact dermatitis (irritant and allergic) who stopped being exposed to the contact irritants and allergens were slightly better than in those who continued. The overall clearance rates for patients who stopped was 73% compared to 69% for those who continued. The corresponding rates for allergic contact dermatitis were 71% for workers who stopped and 74% for those who continued, and for those with irritant contact dermatitis the rates were 74 and 68%, respectively [9].

In Sydney, the prognosis was significantly poorer in patients who continued to work (clearance rate 28%) compared to those who changed jobs (clearance rate 43%) [10].

Among construction workers with allergic contact dermatitis from chromates, Halbert et al. [13] reported that 48% of their workers changed their job and after 6 months to 9 years of follow-up, 31% had complete clearance of their dermatitis.

Prognosis and Atopy

A personal history of atopy also appeared to significantly affect the prognosis of patients with occupational contact dermatitis. Rosen and Freeman [10] reported that the clearance rates in patients with atopy (30%) were significantly poorer than in those without atopy (41%). The corresponding figures if one included workers whose dermatitis was graded 'better' were 79 and 62%, respectively.

In contrast, Halbert et al. [13] did not notice any significant difference in prognosis between workers with chromate dermatitis with and without atopic diathesis.

Similarly, Nethercott and Holness [11] did not report any significant difference in prognosis between atopics and nonatopic workers with occupational dermatitis. The clearance rates were 59 and 65%, respectively.

Causes of Chronicity

The causes for chronicity from contact dermatitis are usually multifactorial. Patients with allergic contact dermatitis are less prone to develop chronicity compared to those with irritant contact dermatitis. One reason could be because in allergic contact dermatitis a specific causative contactant can be identified and avoided by the patient. Generally, the more the patient knows about the causative allergen and its sources, the better the prognosis.

Unlike allergic contact dermatitis, the specific cause of irritant contact dermatitis is often unknown. There is often an associated underlying endogenous eczema in patients with irritant contact dermatitis.

The best predictor for chronicity appears to be a past history of atopic eczema, in particular hand eczema. The cause of chronicity for most patients with contact dermatitis is unknown. Possible causes include (a) continued exposure to irritants or allergens which may be either self-inflicted due to psychological causes (e.g. dermatitis artifacta) or from intentional injury for financial gain from compensation; (b) unrecognized concomitant contact irritant contact dermatitis, e.g. from domestic exposures; (c) unrecognized concomitant allergic contact dermatitis, e.g. from topical medication, gloves or barrier creams.

Conclusion

Numerous factors influence the outcome of contact dermatitis. Patients with allergic contact dermatitis (with the exception of chromate allergy) appear to have slighter better prognosis than patients with irritant contact dermatitis. In allergic contact dermatitis, a specific contact allergen can often be identified and patients are advised to avoid it. In irritant contact dermatitis, the cause is often multifactorial. Risk factors include the present and past history of eczema and atopy. Job change tends to improve outcome but many continued to have dermatitis after changing. Most workers prefer not to change their job. Social prognosis has to be taken into consideration when advising patients on job change.

The prognosis of contact dermatitis appears to be better in recent years compared to that reported earlier. The improvement could be due to better understanding of the disease including (a) the indentification of hidden sources of contact irritants and allergens; (b) better diagnostic skills of dermatologists as a result of availability of better diagnostic tools, e.g. patch test allergens; (c) better education enabling patients to understand and follow advice more readily; (d) better health education programme.

References

1 Skog E, Tottie M: Occupational eczema causing disablement. Acta Derm Venereol 1961;41:205–212.
2 Agrup G: Hand eczema and other hand dermatoses in South Sweden. Acta Derm Venereol 1969; 49{suppl):61.
3 Burrows D: Prognosis in industrial dermatitis. Br J Dermatol 1972;87:145–148.
4 Fregert S: Occupational dermatitis in a 10-year material. Contact Dermatitis 1975;1:96–107.

5 Christensen OB: Prognosis in nickel allergy and hand eczema. Contact Dermatitis 1982;8:7–15.
6 Coenraads PJ: Prevalence of hand eczema: Association with occupational exposure, especially in construction workers; thesis, University of Groningen, 1983.
7 Schubert H, Berova N, Czernielewski A, et al: Epidemiology of nickel allergy. Contact Dermatitis 1987;16:122–128.
8 Pryce DW, Irvine D, English JSC, et al: Soluble oil dermatitis: A follow-up study. Contact Dermatitis 1989;21:28–35.
9 Chia SE, Goh CL: Prognosis of occupational dermatitis in Singapore Worker. Am J Contact Dermatitis 1991;2:105–109.
10 Rosen RH, Freeman S: Prognosis of occupational contact dermatitis in New South Wales, Australia. Contact Dermatitis 1993;29:88–93.
11 Nethercott J, Holness L: Disease outcome in workers with occupational skin disease. J Am Acad Dermatol 1994;30:569–574.
12 Avnstorp C: Follow-up of workers from the prefabricated concrete industry after the addition of ferrous sulphate to Danish cement. Contact Dermatitis 1989;20:365–371.
13 Halbert AR, Gebauer KA, Wall LM: Prognosis of occupational chromate dermatitis. Contact Dermatitis 1992;27:214–219.
14 Matsunaga K, Hosokawa K, Suzuki M, Arima Y, Hayakawa R: Occupational allergic contact dermatitis in beautician. Contact Dermatitis 1988;18:94–96.
15 Rystedt I: Hand eczema and long-term prognosis in atopic dermatitis. Acta Derm Venereol 1985; 117(suppl):1–59.
16 Hellier FF: The prognosis in industrial dermatitis. Br Med J 1958;1:196–198.
17 Keczkes K, Bhate SM, Wyatt EH: The outcome of primary irritant hand dermatitis. Br J Dermatol 1983;109:665–668.
18 Williamson KS: A prognostic study of occupational dermatitis cases in a chemical works. Br J Industr Med 1967;24:103.
19 Hjorth N, Avnstorp C: Rehabilitation in hand eczema. Dermatosen 1986;34:74–76.

Dr. C.L. Goh, Institute of Dermatology, Singapore National Skin Centre,
Singapore 1130 (Singapore)

Elsner P, Lachapelle JM, Wahlberg JE, Maibach HI (eds): Prevention of Contact Dermatitis. Curr Probl Dermatol. Basel, Karger, 1996, vol 25, pp 163–169

Barrier Effect of Gloves against Cytostatic Drugs

Gunh A. Mellström[a, b], *Siv Johansson*[a], *Eva Nyhammar*[a]

[a] Central Laboratory, The National Corporation of Swedish Pharmacies, Stockholm;
[b] Department of Occupational Dermatology, National Institute for Working Life, Solna, Sweden

Cytostatic drugs have potent pharmacological properties and can cause acute skin injuries in cases of accidental exposure. The extent of health hazard due to chronic exposure to small amounts of cytostatic drugs during handling is still not completely known and it is therefore necessary to minimise the exposure. When preparing, dispensing and administering these drugs and standard procedures, the appropriate technique together with protective gloves should be used. The aim of the present study was to investigate the barrier effect of the different gloves recommended for use when preparing cytostatic drugs in the hospital pharmacies and production units of the National Corporation of Swedish Pharmacies.

Materials and Methods

Four brands of medical glove for single use, of three different materials, natural rubber latex, polyvinylchloride (PVC) and ethylmethacrylate; (EMA) were continuously exposed to the cytostatic preparations for 180 min (table 1). The agents tested represented preparations with different chemical structures and modes of action (bleomycin, carmustine, cyclophosphamide, etoposide, mitoxantrone) (table 2). Latex gloves pretreated for 10 min with 70% ethanol were also tested. Those preparations that permeated the latex gloves were subsequently tested with double gloves (latex/PVC and latex/EMA).

The breakthrough times and permeation rates were determined according to the European Standard test method: Protection against liquid chemicals; Resistance of materials to permeation by liquids (EN 396). In this standard, the breakthrough time is defined as the time elapsing from first contact to the point when the measured permeation rate has reached 1 μg/cm^2 min. A two-chamber permeation cell made of stainless steel as required by the

Table 1. Medical gloves for single use

Name	Material	Thickness mm	Supplier
Sempermed Protector™	natural rubber latex	0.32	Selefatrade AB
Ansell NuTex™	natural rubber latex	0.21	Ansell Medical
Evercare™	vinyl (PVC)	0.15	Selefatrade AB
Medette™	EMA plastic	0.03	Triplus AB

Table 2. Preparations of cytostatic drugs

Preparation/ trade name	Generic name	MW	Concentration	Solvent
Alkaloids				
Vepecid®	etoposide	589	20 mg/ml	benzyl alcohol, ethanol
Antibiotics				
Bleomycin	bleomycin	1400	5 IU/ml	NaCl solution
Novantrone®	mitoxantrone	517	2 mg/ml	water
Alkylating drugs				
Cyklofosfamide	cylcophos-phamide	279	20 mg/ml	water
Becenun®	carmustine	214	3.3 mg/ml	ethanol, water

standard was used in a closed-loop system with water as collecting medium. A circular piece from the palm of the glove was mounted in the test cell with the glove outside in contact with the cytostatic preparation and the inside against the collecting medium. Samples for analysis were taken after 5, 10, 30, 60, 90 and 180 min of continuous exposure. The concentration of permeated drugs was determined by HPLC methods.

Results

For the preparations bleomycin, cyclophosphamide, etoposide and mitoxantrone, no breakthrough times were registered or any traces of the drugs detected after 180 min. Only the carmustine preparation permeated some of

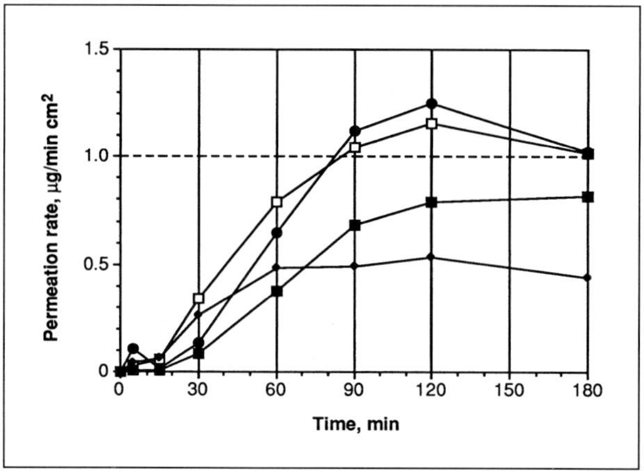

Fig. 1. Permeation of carmustine through gloves of latex 0.32 mm (■), latex 0.21 mm (□), vinyl 0.15 mm (●), EMA plastic 0.03 mm (♦).

the glove materials to the breakthrough time level (1 µg/cm^2 min). For the thin latex glove and the PVC glove, traces of carmustine were detected already after 5 min but breakthrough times were not registered until 60–90 min (fig. 1). Double gloves increased the barrier effect and treatment with 70% ethanol for 10 min did affect the resistance of the glove mateiral (figs. 2, 3).

In the blank tests of the latex gloves and the solvents used in the preparations of etoposide and bleomycin there were indications that some rubber chemical agents leached from the glove material itself.

Discussion

The introduction of special guidelines and safety precautions for handling cytostatic drugs started more than 10 years ago in several countries [2–7]. To minimise the exposure when preparing, dispensing and administering these drugs, standard procedures, appropriate technique together with personal protective equipment, e.g. gloves, should be used. However, there are no requirements or criteria for evaluating medical glove quality for protection against permeation by hazardous agents. Today, the quality control of medical gloves is mainly restricted to leakage testing. A standard for single-use medical gloves with requirements of labelling and biocompatibility is being developed in the CEN (Committee for European Normalisation) TC 205/WG3. The standard methods available for testing permeation by hazardous chemicals are required

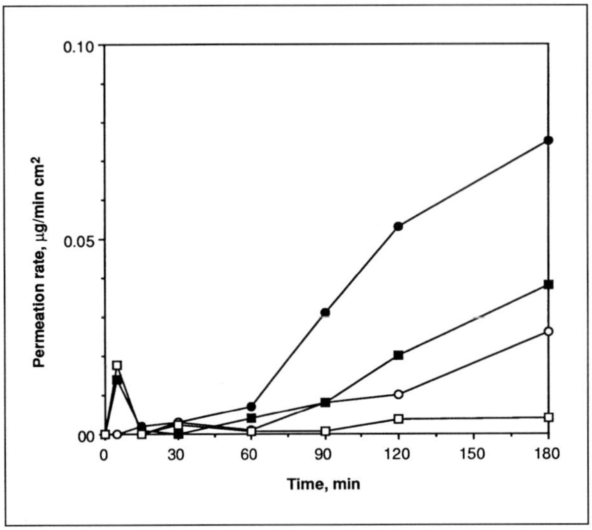

Fig. 2. Permeation of carmustine through double gloves. ● = Latex 0.21/vinyl 0.15 min, ○ = latex 0.21/EMA-plastic 0.03 mm; ■ = latex 0.32/vinyl 0.15 min; □ = latex 0.32/EMA-plastic 0.03 mm.

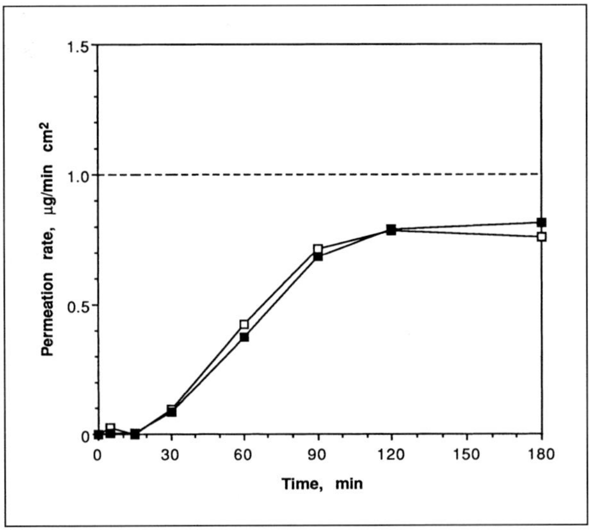

Fig. 3. Permeation of carmustine through latex gloves 0.32 mm. ■ = Untreated; □ = pretreated with 70% ethanol.

for establishing the barrier resistance capacity of protective gloves but not for medical gloves for single use (which are classified as medical devices and not personal protective equipment) [1, 8].

Test data on the barrier effect of protective clothing, gloves included, to permeation by chemicals are available in databases and guideline books. But data concerning cytotoxic drugs are uncommon in these sources, probably because medical gloves are not defined as protective gloves [9, 11]. Although there are reports on the permeability of gloves by several cytostatic drugs, the procedures used are not standardised and the analytical methods, equipment and sensitivity diverge tremendously, and therefore the test results are hard to compare and evaluate. In a permeation study by Mader et al. [12] with 12 cytostatic drugs tested with one brand of latex glove, one conclusion was that the drugs could be divided into three groups; nonpermeating drugs (>4 h), slowly permeating drugs (after 2 h but not 4 h) and rapidly permeating drugs (<15 min). Three factors seem to crucially affect the permeation through the lipophilic natural latex glove membrane: pH value (ionisation), lipophilicity and molecular size. Even gloves intended for handling cytostatic drugs are permeated by carmustine within 10–15 min [13, 14]. In another study, 23 different brands of natural rubber latex and plastic glove were tested against carmustine with breakthrough times varying from 5 to 60 min due to different material thickness and barrier capacity [15]. The need for requirements for barrier effect against hazardous drugs for medical gloves has recently been shown by Sessink et al. [16]. They studied occupational exposure to cyclophosphamide, 5-fluoruracil and methotrexate in technicians involved in drug preparation. Contamination and permeation through latex gloves were found for each of the three compounds [16].

Today some medical gloves are offered for use in handling cytostatic drugs, these should fulfil the permeation requirements for protective gloves, and not only the leakage requirements for medical gloves. Hence, they should be labelled with a protection index for the specific drugs they are intended to give protection against [17, 18]. In the present study the EN standard method for testing resistance of *protective clothing* to permeation was chosen, as at that time a draft standard method for permeation testing *protective gloves* (prEN) had not yet been adopted by the EU member countries as an EN Standard Method [1, 8, 17]. The performance of the two permeation methods is quite similar. The permeation test cells are different but this has little influence on the determination of breakthrough time [18]. In these two standard methods the breakthrough time is defined as the time elapsing from the first contact and the point when the permeation rate has reached 1 μg/min cm^2. This definition facilitates and improves comparison of the test results as the results are less dependent on what technical equipment is used and on analytical sensitivity. In our study detectable amounts of carmustine were found already after 5 min but the permeation rate was very low and the level of 1 μg/min cm^2 was not reached until after 60–90 min. Glove membrane thickness and formulation crucially influence the barrier effect against hazardous agents [19, 20]. This was verified in our study, where the thin glove (0.03 mm) of EMA showed the best resistance to carmustine (fig. 1). It was also evident that double gloves increase the barrier effect (fig. 2). The present results also indicated that a short pretreatment with 70% ethanol had no influence on the barrier effect of the glove material, but that alcoholic solvents can contribute to the leaching of rubber chemical from natural rubber latex. The manufacturers of the two latex gloves confirmed that both brands of latex glove contained zinc dithiocarbamate (ZDC) and one brand also mercaptobenzothiazol (MBT). Control tests with the latex gloves and the rubber chemical substances confirmed that these substances leached from the glove material. After contact with an alcoholic solvent the leaching was higher than after contact with an aqueous solvent.

Conclusions

Only carmustine permeated the glove materials at the permeation rate level defined as breakthrough time (1 μg/min cm^2). Double gloves reduced the permeation rate and pretreatment with 70% ethanol for 10 min did not influence the barrier effect of the glove material. Rubber chemicals (ZDC, MBT) leached from the latex gloves. The gloves tested will provide acceptable protection for 3 h when working with bleomycine, cyclophosphamide, etoposide and mitoxantrone and similar drug preparations. Working with carmustine preparations, gloves should be replaced as soon as possible after accidental exposure. To avoid side effects caused by latex gloves and to improve the resistance to permeation of cytostatic drugs, latex gloves with inner gloves of PVC or EMA are recommended.

References

1 SS-European Standard EN 369: Protective clothing – protection against chemicals – test method: Resistance of materials to permeation by liquids. Brussels, European Committee for Standardisation, 1994.

2 Knowles RS, Virden JE: Occasional review: Handling of injectable antineoplastic agents. Br Med J 1980;30:589–591.

3 Anon: Guidelines Concerning the Handling of Cytostatic Agents. Norway, Directorate of Labour Inspection, 1980.

4 Anon: Guidelines for the Handling of Hazardous Pharmaceuticals. Toronto, Canadian Society of Hospital Pharmacists, 1981.

5 Anon: Guidelines Concerning the Handling of Cytostatic Agents. Stockholm, Swedish National Board of Occupational Safety and Health, 1984, p 8.
6 Anon: OSHA work-practice guidelines for personnel dealing with cytotoxic (antineoplastic) drugs. Am J Hosp Pharm 1986;43:1193–1204.
7 Anon: ASHP Technical Assistance Bulletin on Handling Cytotoxic and Hazardous Drugs. Am J Hosp Pharm 1990;4:1033–1049.
8 SS-European Standard EN 374–1: Protective Gloves against Chemicals and Micro-organisms, 3. Determination of Resistance to Permeation by Chemicals. Brussels, European Committee for Standardisation, 1994.
9 Schwope AD, Costas PP, Jackson JO, Weitzman JO: Guidelines for the Selection of Protective Clothing. Cincinnati, American Conference of Governmental Industrial Hygienists, Inc (2nd), 1985.
10 Mellström GA: Information sources for glove test data; in Mellström GA, Wahlberg JE, Maibach HI (eds): Protective Gloves for Occupational Use. Boca Raton, CRC Press, 1994, pp 293–303.
11 Forsberg K, Keith LH: Chemical Protective Clothing: Permeation and Degradation Compendium. Boca Raton, Lewis Publishers, 1995.
12 Mader RM, Rizovski B, Steger GG, Moser K, Rainer H, Dittrich C: Permeability of latex membranes to anti-cancer drugs. Int J Pharm 1991;68:151–156.
13 Dinter-Heidorn H, Carstens G: Comparative study on protective gloves for handling cytotoxic medicaments: A model study with carmustine. Pharm Weekblad Sci Ed 1992;4:180–184.
14 Stjernström G, Landersjö L, Angdin B: Permeation of antineoplastic agents through surgical gloves. 1st Scand Symp Protective Clothing against Chemicals and Other Health Risks, Copenhagen, 1984 (abstract). Copenhagen, NOKOBETEF, c/o HAZARPREVENT.
15 Thomas PH, Fenton-May V: Protection offered by various gloves to carmustine exposure. Pharm J 1987;20:775–777.
16 Sessink PJM, van de Kerkhof MCA, Anzion RB, Bos RP: Environmental contaminationa and assessment of exposure to antineoplastic agents by determination of cyclophosphamide in urine of exposed pharmacy technicians: Is skin absorption an important exposure route? Arch Envir Health 1994;4:165–169.
17 Meddström GA, Carlsson B: European standards on protective gloves; in Mellström GA, Wahlberg JE, Maibach HI (eds): Protective Gloves for Occupational Use Boca Raton, CRC Press, 1994, pp 39–43.
18 Mellström GA, Carlsson B, Boman AS: Testing of protective effect against liquid chemicals; in Mellström GA, Wahlberg JE, Maibach HI (eds): Protective Gloves for Occupational Use. Boca Raton, CRC Press, 1994, pp 53–77.
19 Mickelsen RL, Hall RC: A breakthrough time comparison of nitrile and neoprene glove materials produced by different glove manufacturers. Am Ind Hyg Assoc J 1987;48:941–947.
20 Sansone EB, Tewari YB: Differences in the extent of solvent penetration through natural rubber and nitrile gloves from various manufacturers. Am Ind Hyg Assoc J 1980;41:527–528.

Dr. Gunh A. Mellström, LUPS, Build 211:3, Pharmaceutical and Analytical R&D,
Astra Pain Control AB, S–151 85 Södertälje (Sweden)

Elsner P, Lachapelle JM, Wahlberg JE, Maibach HI (eds): Prevention of Contact Dermatitis. Curr Probl Dermatol. Basel, Karger, 1996, vol 25, pp 170–176

Rubber Glove Dermatitis: A Significant Occupational Hazard-Prevention

T. Estlander, R. Jolanki, L. Kanerva

Finnish Institute of Occupational Helath, Section of Dermatology, Helsinki, Finland

Protective gloves made of polymeric rubber or plastic materials are important safeguards against factors hazardous to hands. But their use entails many problems of which the development of allergy, especially to rubber glove materials and other possible agents used in gloves, is probably the most harmful [1, 2].

Two Forms of Allergic Reactions Caused by Rubber Gloves

Two forms of allergic reactions to rubber gloves prevail: delayed (type IV allergy), and immediate (type I allergy). Since the 1930s gloves have been reported to evoke delayed allergy to rubber [2] whereas the first cases of immediate allergy to natural rubber latex (NRL) gloves were reported in the late 1970s [3, 4]. Since then hundreds of new cases of type I allergy to NRL, mostly in connection with the use of gloves, have been published [5]. Most of the reported cases of type IV allergy to rubber gloves are due to gloves made of NRL [2, 6]. Reports on cases due to synthetic materials are few, and usually describe allergy to neoprene rubber gloves [2, 7, 8], but sensitization to other materials, e.g. nitrile rubber, is also possible [8]. All reported cases of type I allergy have been caused by NRL gloves [5].

Clinical Symptoms of Rubber Glove Allergy

Both types of rubber glove allergy are signalled by a skin inflammation mainly on the hands and wrists. A typical symptom of type I allergy to NRL gloves is contact urticaria, but the symptoms can consist of itching and redness of the skin only or aggravation of the pre-existing dermatitis. They can also include generalized urticaria, conjunctivitis, rhinitis, and asthma, or appear as serious anaphylactic reactions [5, 9, 10]. Delayed allergic reactions are generally confined to the skin. Eczematous lesions appear on the site covered by the glove, but forearms and even larger areas including the face may also be involved. Glove allergy usually involves one of the two types of reactions, but occasionally both coincide [5, 9, 10].

Sensitizers in Rubber Gloves

The primary ingredient in rubber gloves is rubber polymer which is blended with accelerators, antioxidants, pigments, fillers and other additives. Rubber polymer can be made from the milky liquid (natural latex) of the rubber tree, or manufactured synthetically. Whether a rubber glove is called natural (NRL) or synthetic depends on the type of polymer used in its production. Neoprene and nitrile rubbers are examples of synthetic materials. Blending NRL with neoprene or nitrile rubbers is also a common practice [2, 9, 11].

Additives, usually accelerators such as thiurams, carbamates and benzothiazoles and antioxidants are responsible for type IV allergy due to gloves [2, 6, 9, 10]. Other potential type IV sensitizers in rubber gloves include other chemicals, e.g. thiourea and phenol derivatives, diphenylguanidine, mercaptobenzimidazole, quinoline derivatives, vulcanizers, colorants, preservatives, antistatic agents, glove powder ingredients as well as fragrances [2, 9, 10, 12]. Rubber polymer itself has also long been listed as a possible cause of delayed allergy to rubber [2, 13].

Thiurams and carbamates are frequently used in gloves. Correspondingly, thiurams have most commonly been responsible for the reactions due to rubber gloves. Carbamates are the second most common cause of type IV allergic reactions in glove allergic patients [2, 6, 9, 10, 14]. Mercaptobenzothiazole was the first benzothiazole accelerator used in gloves, but other derivatives can also be included [2, 9, 11]. The reports on sensitization to thiourea compounds from rubber gloves [2, 7, 8] are few. Diphenylthiourea is one of such chemicals used in neoprene gloves [7].

Antioxidants are less frequent sensitizers in gloves [2, 9]. Sensitization from gloves to N-isopropyl-N-phenyl-PPDA (paraphenylenediamine) have been published [2, 9, 14], although PPDA derivatives are seldom used in rubber gloves except in black or dark-colored industrial gloves. Phenol derivatives, e.g. dihydroxydiphenyl, have only rarely induced sensitization [2, 9].

Proteins in NRL polymers [5] are the chief cause of type I allergy, whereas casein [15] and terpenes [16] may also be possible allergens. Other potential sensitizers include additives of rubber mixtures (e.g. thiurams, carbamates) [9, 10, 17] and protein impurities in glove powders [10]. Recently, certain polyurethane-coated surgical NRL gloves have been reported as a new possible cause of glove contact urticaria, probably from NRL in the glove material [18].

Proteins with molecular weight (MW) ranging from 14 to 75 kD are usually responsible for allergy to NRL, but allergenic proteins may also have a lower or higher MW [19]. In addition, the manufacturing process of the gloves may cause some of the proteins to become even more allergenic [20]. Glove brands also vary greatly in allergenicity: some sensitized persons may even be able to use NRL gloves with low allergenicity [21]. Hamann [22] has reviewed factors affecting antigenicity and the concentration of NRL proteins.

Rubber Gloves as Sources of Occupational Allergy

Rubber gloves are considered to be the main source of occupational allergy to rubber [2, 9, 10, 14], 41–66% of all occupationally induced type IV rubber allergy cases have been reported to be caused by rubber gloves [2, 6, 23, 24]. Even higher figures (95–96%) for gloves as causes of occupational rubber sensitization have been reported when housewives are included in the occupational groups [25, 26]. Allergy to gloves seems to be especially frequent among women, but it is also common among male workers who regularly use rubber gloves [2, 9, 10, 27]. Long-standing use of rubber gloves, and simultaneous exposure of the hands to chemical or mechanical irritants or wet work seems to constitute the most important risk of developing type IV allergy to gloves. Risk occupations include work in medical and dental health services, laboratory work, cleaning, hair dressing, kitchen work or work in the food industries, farm house work, and industrial work [2, 9, 10]. In a recent follow-up study of occupational contact allergy to rubber chemicals [23], 85% of the patients worked in such occupations. Of industrial workers, masons [25] and construction workers [14] have been reported to be the most common occupations entailing risk of rubber glove allergy.

Rubber gloves are an important cause of NRL allergy, although there are also many other sources of NRL contact [5, 9, 10, 22]. In addition to the frequent use of NRL gloves, atopic constitution and hand eczema have often been connected with allergy to NRL [5, 9, 10]. Type I sensitization to NRL gloves is most frequent among hospital and dental care employees, ranging from 2.9 to 14.2%, but it is also common in other occupations where RNL

Table 1. Contact urticaria/protein contact dermatitis (n = 814), Finnish Register of Occupational Diseases (ROD) 1990–1994

Case	n	%
Organic materials	560	69
Natural rubber	193	23
Foods	25	3
Chemicals	14	2
Other	22	3
Total	814	100

Table 2. Allergic contact eczema (n = 1,932), Finnish Register of Occupational Diseases (ROD) 1990–1994

Cause	n	%
Rubber chemicals	508	26
Plastics	367	19
Metals	297	15
Aldehydes	112	6
Other	589	31
Unknown	59	3
Total	1,932	100

gloves are worn daily for long periods [5, 9, 10, 19, 27]. Since 1985 there has been remarkable worldwide increase in the reported cases of type I allergy to NRL gloves [10, 22].

An increase in the occupationally induced cases of allergy to NRL gloves has also been found in Finland. 111 cases of rubber glove dermatoses were diagnosed during 1974–1991 at the Finnish Institute of Occupational Health (FIOH) [2]. 88% of these cases were allergic contact eczema and only 12% were contact urticaria. During the past 5 years a clear increase in the proportion of type I sensitization to NRL gloves can, however, be observed based on the information obtained from the Finnish Register of Occupational Diseases (ROD). During 1990–1994, 814 new cases of contact urticaria and protein contact dermatitis were reported to the ROD (table 1). Natural rubber (193 cases) was the second most common cause of these dermatoses and was responsible for 23% of the cases. Gloves made of NRL caused practically all these cases. 43 of 193 cases of type I NRL allergy were recorded in the ROD in the years 1990 and 1991, whereas in 1992–1993 there were already as many as 96 cases. In 1994 alone the number of reported new cases was 54. In the same period (table 2) rubber chemicals were the most important cause of allergic contact eczema, explaining 26% of the cases. Rubber gloves were considered to be the most common source of type IV allergy to rubber chemicals. When all occupations were concerned, type IV allergy to rubber gloves was, however, more common than type I allergy. Roughly 60% of the glove allergy cases were due to a reaction of delayed type and 40% to an immediate-type reaction. In certain occupations where NRL gloves are used for long periods a day, type I allergy can probably be more important than type IV allergy [27]. Rubber gloves can still be considered the main cause of occupational allergy to rubber. They are responsible for more than half of the occupationally related cases of rubber allergy in Finland. NRL gloves are the most problematic source of rubber allergy; they are a common cause of both type I and type IV allergy.

Prevention

All efforts are necessary to minimize the role of protective gloves as a cause of occupationally induced sensitization to rubber, and to prevent the long-lasting occupational and social consequences of the allergy [23]. Some important aspects of prevention are given below [1, 2].

A detailed job analysis and checking of all materials to be handled with the gloves are always necessary to see whether the glove material is suitable for the job in question. Chemicals coming into contact with rubber glove materials may even promote the development of allergy to the glove ingredients, e.g. organic solvents can extract allergenic compounds from the gloves and carry them inside the gloves [28, 29], some other chemicals, e.g. hypochlorite, can transform a nonallergenic chemical in a rubber material so that it becomes allergenic [30]. The allergenity of the glove may also depend on other environmental factors, e.g. whether the glove is used in an oxidizing or a reducing milieu [31].

The workers need detailed instructions on the use and care of the gloves. In addition, each work place needs to establish good glove care and a control program. Only gloves clearly marked as to the material content should be used [1, 32].

The European directives on personal protective equipment (PPE) (89/686/EEC and 89/656/EEC) already in force in EU countries will possibly affect positively on some aspects regarding the use of gloves. Since July 1, 1995 only PPE with the CE mark can be distributed inside the European Economic Area. This mark guarantees that the product fulfils the essential requirements of Directive 89/686/EEC. It also implies that the CE mark can be given only by some of the notified EU bodies, e.g. the Department of Physics of FIOH in Finland. Directive 89/656/EEC obligates employers to make risk assessments and define the suitability of gloves for each job, as well as to organize a system of glove maintenance and training for glove users.

It is also important that rubber gloves are not used needlessly. Their use should be avoided for instance during cleaning jobs in which no liquids are handled. The use of polymer gloves should be started at the same time as the handling of hazardous materials; one should not wait until the skin is inflamed and the barrier broken. All polymer gloves are designed to protect intact healthy skin. No glove offers an instant solution to the problem of hand dermatitis. Gloves should be used only temporarily to protect inflamed skin [1].

Gloves made of plastic or synthetic rubber materials should be primarily used for hand protection when constant use of polymer gloves is necessary. Especially plastic materials rarely cause allergic dermatitis [2], but their prolonged use carries the same risk of maceration as rubber gloves. When the use of rubber gloves is necessary, the best choice is to use gloves made of synthetic rubber worn with inner cotton gloves. NRL gloves are best for occasional use. Inner cotton or inner disposable PVC or PE (polyethylene) gloves are recommended to be used with NRL gloves, because the inner gloves increase the protection of the gloves and decrease the risk of sensitization to the glove material [1, 2].

Despite the risk of allergy, NRL and other rubber gloves still retain their place as effective means of protection provided that they are used correctly and chosen for the right jobs. There is, however, a need of NRL gloves from which as many sensitizing proteins as possible have been eliminated and the amount of allergenic additives has been minimized. The development of standards to define the contents of gloves with low allergenity has already been started by the European Committee for Standardization (CEN), e.g. the standard concerning disposable medical gloves ('medical gloves for single' use) is under preparation by a working group (CEN/TC 205/WG3) with, e.g., Finnish and Swedish experts on NRL allergy as its members.

References

1 Estlander T, Jolanki R: How to protect the hands. Dermatol Clin 1988;5:105–114.

2 Estlander T, Jolanki R, Kanerva L: Allergic contact dermatitis from rubber and plastic gloves, in Mellström GA, Wahlberg JE, Maibach HI (eds): Protective Gloves for Occupational Use. Boca Raton, CRC Press, 1994, pp 221–239.

3 Nutter AF: Contact urticaria to rubber. Br J Dermatol 1979;101:597–598.

4 Förström L: Contact urticaria from latex surgical gloves. Contact Dermatitis 1980;6:33–34.

5 Turjanmaa K: Contact urticaria from latex gloves; in Mellström GA, Wahlberg JE, Maibach HI (eds): Protective Gloves for Occupational Use. Boca Raton, CRC Press, 1994, pp 241–254.

6 Heese A, von Hintzenstern J, Peters K-P, Koch HU, Hornstein OP: Allergic and irritant reactions to rubber gloves in medical health services. J Am Acad Dermatol 1991;25:831–839.

7 Kanerva L, Estlander T, Jolanki R: Occupational allergic contact dermatitis caused by thiourea compounds. Contact Dermatitis 1994;31:242–248.
8 Estlander T, Kanerva L, Jolanki R: Rubber additive sensitization from synthetic rubber gloves and boots. Allergologie 1995;18:470.
9 Fuchs T: Gummi und Allergie. München-Deisenhofen, Dustri, 1995, pp 1–247.
10 Heese A, Peters K-P, Koch HU, Hornstein OP: Allergien gegen Latexhandschuhe. Allergologie 1995;18:358–365.
11 Mellström GA, Boman A: Gloves: Types, materials, and manufacturing; in Mellström GA, Wahlberg JE, Maibach HI (eds): Protective Gloves for Occupational Use. Boca Raton, CRC Press, 1994, pp 21–35.
12 Cronin E: Rubber; in: Contact Dermatitis. Edinburgh, Churchill-Livingstone 1980, pp 714–770.
13 Wyss M, Elsner P, Wütrich B, Burg G: Allergic contact dermatitis from natural latex without contact urticaria. Contact Dermatitis 1993;28:154–156.
14 Conde-Salazar L, del-Rio E, Guimaraens D, Domingo AG: Type IV allergy to rubber additives: A 10-year study of 686 cases. J Am Acad Dermatol 1993;29:176–180.
15 Mäkinen-Kiljunen S, Reunala T, Turjanmaa K, Cacioli P: Is cows' milk casein an allergen in latex-rubber gloves? Lancet 1993;342:863–864.
16 Seaton A, Cherrie B, Turnbull J: Rubber glove asthma. Br Med J 1988;296:531–532.
17 Belsito DV: Contact urticaria caused by rubber. Dermatol Clin 1990;8:61–66.
18 Kwangsukstith CH, Maibach HI: Contact urticaria from polyurethane-membrane hypoallergenic gloves. Contact Dermatitis 1995;33:200–201.
19 Mäkinen-Kiljunen S, Turjanmaa K: Latexallergene in verschiedenen Arten von Latex-Handschuhen und Sensibilisierung von Krankenhauspersonal und Patienten. Allergologie 1995;18:366–368.
20 Alenius H, Turjanmaa K, Palosuo T, Mäkinen-Kiljunen S, Reunala T: Surgical latex glove allergy: Characterization of rubber protein allergens by immunoblotting. Int Arch Allergy Appl Immunol 1991;96:376–380.
21 Cormio L, Turjanmaa K, Talja M, Andersson LC, Ruutu M: Toxicity and immediate allergenicity of latex gloves. Clin Exp Allergy 1993;23:618–623.
22 Hamann CP: Natural rubber latex protein sensitivity in review. Am J Contact Dermatitis 1993;4:4–21.
23 Wrangsjö K, Meding B: Occupational allergy to rubber chemicals: A follow-up study. Dermatosen 1994;42:184–189.
24 Estlander T: Occupatinal skin disease in Finland: Observations made during 1974–1988 at the Institute of Occupational Health, Helsinki (thesis). Acta Derm Venereol 1990;(suppl 155):1–71.
25 Romaguera C, Grimalt F: Statistical and comparative study of 4600 patients tested in Barcelona (1973–1977). Contact Dermatitis 1980;6:309–315.
26 Themido R, Menezes Brandao F: Contact allergy to thiurams. Contact Dermatitis 1984;10:251.
27 Tarvainen K, Jolanki R, Forsman-Grönholm L, Estlander T, Pfäffli P, Juntunen J, Kanerva L: Exposure, skin protection and occupational skin diseases in the glass fibre reinforced plastics industry. Contact Dermatitis 1993;29:119–127.
28 Williams JR: Permeation of glove materials by physiologically harmful chemicals. Am Ind Hyg Assoc J 1979;40:877–882.
29 Estlander T, Kilpikari I, Eskolin E: Polymeerikäsineen läpäisevyys ja sen valmistuksessa käytettävät kemikaalit (Permeability of polymer gloves and chemicals used in the manufacture of gloves). Suomen Lääkärilehti (Finnish Med J) 1980;35:800–803.
30 Jordan WP, Bourlas MC: Allergic contact dermatitis to underwear elastic, chemically transformed by a laundry bleach. Arch Dermatol 1975;111:593–595.
31 Hanson C, Ågrup G: Stability of mercaptobenzothiazole compounds. Contact Dermatitis 1993;28:29–34.
32 Estlander T, Jolanki R, Kanerva L: Contact urticaria from rubber gloves: A detailed description of four cases. Acta Derm Venereol 1987;134:98–102.

Tuula Estlander, MD, PhD, Finnish Institute of Occupational Health,
Section of Occupational Dermatology, Topeliuksenkatu 41 a A, FIN–00250 Helsinki (Finland)

Elsner P, Lachapelle JM, Wahlberg JE, Maibach HI (eds): Prevention of Contact Dermatitis. Curr Probl Dermatol. Basel, Karger, 1996, vol 25, pp 177–181

European Standards on Protective Gloves

Traugott Zimmerli

EMPA Swiss Federal Laboratories for Materials Testing and Research, St. Gallen, Switzerland

The need of having standardized test methods and performance requirements for protective gloves has been recognized for a long time. The users of protective gloves need to be certain that they are protected and they want to know how far they are protected. The manufacturers want to show the users that their product fulfils their needs of protection. And the test laboratories want to have approved and standardized test methods in order to get reproducible results. Standards are developed by different bodies. There are several national standards bodies like AFNOR, ANSI, BSI, DIN and SNV. Then there are regional standards bodies; for Europe it is the European Committee for Standardization CEN. And finally there is the International Organization for Standardization ISO.

When speaking about European standards and in order to understand the special position of these standards, we have to look at the EEC Treaty from 1957 with its amendments introduced in the single European Act from 1986. In article 8a the establishment of the single European market until the end of 1992 is postulated:

> The community takes the necessary measures for the step-by-step realization of the internal market. The internal market comprises an area without internal frontiers, inside which the free exchange of goods, persons, services and capital is guaranteed.

And in article 100a the rules for the functioning of the European market are laid down:

> The Council issues measures (i.e. directives) for the approximation of the laws of the member states which have for subject the establishment and functioning of the internal market.

Directives have been established since then, especially in those fields where it is necessary to maintain a certain performance level of the products which are allowed to freely circulate inside the European market. These are mainly products which are related to occupational and consumer safety, e.g. machine safety, manual handling of loads, gas valves, safety signs at workplace, medical devices and personal protective equipment. The last two will be discussed later in more detail. All products which fulfil the basic safety requirements of the directives may be certified to bear the CE mark, which is not – as many people think – a quality mark, but only a sign which confirms the compliance with the directive. Very soon it has been recognized that it is not possible to lay down all the technical details about the products in the directives and accordingly in the laws of the member states. Therefore, the European Council decided in 1985 to handle the problem according to the so-called 'New approach'. What are the principles of the New Approach? Only the basic safety requirements in very general terms are included in the New Approach directives. These directives have to be implemented into the laws of the member countries. The detailed technical specifications of the products are laid down in the harmonized European standards. Mandates are given to CEN to develop these standards. They remain what they have been since ever, namely voluntary standards. But, products which are tested according to them are assumed to fulfil the essential requirements of the corresponding directive and may therefore bear the CE mark. This explains the very strong position of the standards produced by CEN for the European market.

In the following two of the New Approach directives and the standards on protective gloves based on the essential requirements of these directives will be discussed in more datail. The first is the so-called PPE (personal protective equipment) directive, the 'Council Directive of 21 December 1989 on the approximation of the laws of the Member States relating to personal protective equipment (89/686/EEC)'. In article 1 of this directive a PPE is defined as:

> Any device or appliance designed to be worn or held by an individual for protection against one or more health and safety hazards.

The directive applies to all sorts of PPE except those covered by other directives and some special types of PPE listed in annex I of the directive (e.g. PPE for military, police and self-defence use). The PPE are divided into three catagories, for which different procedures for the certification process are applied.

Category I includes PPE of simple design, protecting against minimal risks which can be safely identified by the user in good time. For this category a self-declaration by the manufacturer that he has fulfilled the essential requirements of the directive is sufficient for the CE marking of the product. PPE of complex design, protecting against serious and mortal danger, which the user cannot identify in sufficient time, is classified in category III. All the rest of the PPE belongs to category II. For the CE marking of the products in categories II and III a type examination by a notified body is necessary and in addition for category III a quality control system or a regular control of the production is necessary. Chemical protective gloves are classified in category III, excluding those for medical use in the patient's environment, for which the medical device directive applies. This directive will be discussed later.

The essential requirements for gloves for protection against dangerous substances and infective agents in cutaneous contact are given in clause 3.10.2 of annex II of the PPE directive:

> PPE intended to prevent the surface contact of all or part of the body with dangerous substances and infective agents must be capable of preventing the penetration or diffusion of such substances through the protective integument under the foreseeable conditions of use for which the PPE is placed on the market.
>
> To this end, the constituent materials and other components of these PPE classes must be so chosen, or designed and incorporated as to ensure, as far as possible, complete leak-tightness, which will allow where necessary prolonged daily use or, failing this, limited leak-tightness necessitating a restriction of the period of wear.
>
> Where, by virtue of their nature and the foreseeable conditions of their use, certain dangerous substances or infective agents possess high penetrative power which limits the duration of the protection provided by the PPE in question, the latter must be subjected to standard tests with a view to their classification on the basis of efficiency. PPE which is considered to be in conformity with the test specifications must bear a mark indicating, in particular, the names or, failing this, the codes of the substances used in the tests and the corresponding standard period of protection. The manufacturer's notes must also contain, in particular, an explanation of the codes (if necessary), a detailed description of the standard tests and all appropriate information for the determination of the maximum permissible period of wear under the different foreseeable conditions of use.

European standards on gloves under the PPE directive have been developed in the Working Group 8 'Hand protection' of the CEN Technical Committee 162 'Protective clothing including hand and arm protection and lifejackets'. In EN 420 general requirements for gloves are specified, which are design principles, glove construction, high-visibility gloves, innocuousness of protective gloves, cleaning, sizing, dexterity and water vapor transmission/absorption.

In the three existing parts of EN 374, the specific requirements for protective gloves against chemicals and microorganisms are laid down. In EN 374-1 'Terminology and performance requirements' the following items are covered: definitions, penetration, permeation, degradation and mechanical characteristics. In EN 374-2 the test methods for the determination of the resistance to penetration are described, which are an air leak test and a water leak test of the complete glove. EN 374-3 describes the test method for the determination of resistance of the glove material to permeation by chemicals. In a standardized test cell the chemical under test is filled on the outer side of the glove material and on the inner side the amount of the chemical permeating through the material is continuously monitored. From the results the breakthrough time and the breakthrough rate is determined. In EN 374-4, which will be issued in the future, a test method for the degradation of gloves will be described.

The second New Approach directive which concerns gloves is the 'Council Directive 93/42/EEC of 14 June 1993 concerning medical devices'. In article 1 the following definitions are given:

> 'Medical device' means any instrument, apparatus, appliance, material or other article, whether used alone or in combination, including the software necessary for its proper application intended by the manufacturer to be used for human beings for the purpose of:
>
> – diagnosis, prevention, monitoring, treatment of alleviation of disease,
> – diagnosis, monitoring, treatment, alleviation of or compensation for an injury or handicap,
> – investigation, replacement or modification of the anatomy or of a physiological process,
> – control of conception,
>
> and which does not achieve its principal intended action in or on the human body by pharmacological, immunological or metabolic means, but which may be assisted in its functions by such means,

and

> 'Device intended for clinical investigation' means any device intended for use by a duly qualified medical practitioner when conducting investigations in an adequate human clinical environment.

This directive covers those gloves which have been excluded from the PPE directive, i.e. gloves for medical use in the patient's environment. The medical device directive is written in a similar way as the PPE directive, but, in contrast to the latter, it focuses more on the safety of the patient and less on that of the wearer of the glove. The medical devices are divided into categories I, IIa, IIb and III according to 18 different rules laid down in annex IX of the directive and, as in the PPE directive, the conformity assessment procedure differs for the different categories.

Standards for gloves are developed in the Working Group 3 'Medical gloves' of the CEN Technical Committee 205 'Non-active medical devices'. There are three parts of EN 455 'Medical gloves for single use'. In EN 455-1 'Requirements and testing for freedom from holes' the same test method as in EN 374-2, the water leak test, is described. In EN 455-2 requirements and test methods for the following physical properties are given: length, width, force to break before accelerated ageing, force to break after accelerated ageing and seam strength of seamed gloves. prEN 455-3 'Requirements and testing for biocompatibility and labelling' is still under development. In the draft the measurement of the contents of leachable proteins and of chemicals as well as the labelling are regulated.

Two other standards which apply also to gloves are under development in CEN/TC 205:

> prEN 1041 'Terminology, symbols and information provided with medical devices – Information supplied by the manufacturer with medical devices'

and

> prEN 1441 'Medical devices – Risk analysis'.

This article gives an overview on the regulations of the single European market, the directives and the special position of the EN standards and explains briefly the existing standards on protective gloves and what prescriptions they make.

Dr. Traugott Zimmerli, Head of Section Clothing/Protective Equipment, EMPA St. Gallen, Lerchenfeldstrasse 5, CH–9014 St. Gallen (Switzerland)

Elsner P, Lachapelle JM, Wahlberg JE, Maibach HI (eds): Prevention of Contact Dermatitis. Curr Probl Dermatol. Basel, Karger, 1996, vol 25, pp 182–192

Efficacy of Protective Creams and/or Gels

J.M. Lachapelle

Unit of Dermato-Allergology and Dermato-Immunology, Laboratory of Occupational and Environmental Dermatology, Catholic University of Louvain, Brussels, Belgium

Protection against environmental hazards is of great concern since handling potentially toxic substances is becoming more and more frequent in occupational and/or domestic life [1].

'Barrier' creams and/or gels are targeted as one of the classical means of skin protection against noxious chemicals from the environment [2]. There has been a lot of controversy concerning their potential efficacy. The qualities which are required for a barrier cream or gel are never entirely fulfilled; therefore, it can be stressed that no 'ideal' protective cream or gel exists at present [3]. A very important rule is to use barrier creams or gels on intact skin only; they have to be considered as tools of primary or secondary prevention and not as treatment measures [4]. It is noteworthy that using protective creams or gels on diseased skin leads unavoidably to increased skin irritation, inducing a deleterious rather than a beneficial effect.

'Active' Protective Creams or Gels Aimed at Preventing Allergic Contact Dermatitis

In former times, 'active' barrier creams have been very popular in some European countries. The term 'active' applies to creams containing active ingredients that are supposed to work by trapping or transforming allergens (ascorbic acid, glutathione, cysteine, ion exchangers, etc.). It has been claimed in recent reviews that they can be considered as ineffective [2]. Indeed, this opinion is broadly expressed by practising dermatologists.

Nevertheless, some recent publications have entertained doubts about this clear-cut view.

Studies are two-sided: (a) application of creams or gels before applying the allergens in a patch test system on the skin of sensitive subjects and evaluation of the reducing effect of the cream or gel on the positive patch test reaction at 24, 48 or 72 h; (b) 'use tests' mimicking real conditions of skin contact with the allergen.

For instance, beneficial results were reported in some chromate-sensitive construction workers using a barrier cream composed of silicone, tartaric acid, glycine and other ingredients. The tartaric acid and glycine apparently chelate chromate and reduce chrome VI to chrome III, which is less allergenic [5].

On the other hand, some compounds offer potential for use in the prophylaxis of nickel dermatitis [6]. Chelating agents and other substances can be used to bind nickel or reduce its penetration through the skin, and hence to reduce the symptoms in subjects with nickel sensitivity. The most effective ligand for nickel so far described is 5-chloro-7-iodoquinolin-8-ol. Although normally regarded as safe, its usage in some situations may be limited by concerns about its toxicity. Other ligands with demonstrable effect include ethylenediamine tetraacetic acid (EDTA) in various forms, diphenylglyoxime and dimethylglyoxime. Cation exchange resins can effectively bind nickel and work both in vitro and in vivo. Propyleneglycol, petrolatum and lanolin reduce absorption of nickel through the skin. In a recent study [7], application of a Carbopol gel with 10% Ca Na_2-EDTA beneath a nickel disc completely abrogated the allergic contact response in 21/21 (100%) nickel-sensitive patients. A Carbopol gel without Ca Na_2-EDTA was less effective, inhibiting the response in 15/21 (71.4%). Further studies are conducted in this direction [8].

Poison ivy/oak (*Toxicodendron*) dermatitis is the most common allergic contact dermatitis in the United States. The allergen is 3-pentadecyl-catechol. Related dermatoses are *Lithrea* dermatitis, commonly encountered in some countries of South America, and lacquer tree dermatitis frequently described mainly in Japan, but also in several countries of East Asia. Until recently, despite extensive research, the use of topical barrier preparations to prevent *Toxicodendron* dermatitis has been only minimally successful.

A very extensive study has been conducted in the United States, in order to find 'active' protective creams and reduce the disability of this quite common skin problem [9]. The results of this study indicate that some barrier creams (Stokogard®, Hollister Moisture Barrier® and Hydropel®) are able to reduce – to a certain extent – the skin symptoms in sensitive subjects. Even more promising is the very recent use of a new topical lotion containing 5% quaternium-18 bentonite [10].

All these trials indicate that new approaches are under current evaluation, but no real consensus can be sorted out nowadays in this difficult and controversial field of research.

'Passive' Protective Creams of Gels Aimed at Preventing Irritant Contact Dermatitis

'Passive' creams or gels correspond to formulations containing no active ingredients such as drugs or chelating agents, but only 'indifferent' ingredients. The aim of such formulations is to shield the horny layer of epidermis by an external 'barrier' of various molecules susceptible to impair the penetration of noxious chemicals from the environment into the skin.

Techniques Used to Assess the Efficacy of Creams or Gels

For a long time critical evaluation of protective creams or gels has been scarce in the literature (fig. 1). In the 1950s Suskind [11] introduced the 'slide test' which is a very simple procedure. It consists of covering a glass slide (of the model used for histological sections) with a thin layer of the formulation under investigation. The slide is then plunged into solutions of various irritants at different concentrations. The 'resistance' of the formulation to the action of the irritants is evaluated. This crude technique does not take into consideration the potential penetration of the irritant through the cream or gel, without eventually affecting its substantiality. In other words, the technique does not preclude the possibility that an irritant solution could be noxious to skin structures without affecting the overlying barrier cream or gel [12–14].

In the late 1970s and early 1980s, some experiments were conducted to study the potential efficacy (or nonefficacy) of barrier formulations on guinea pig or human skin [15, 16]. The skin lesions were evaluated by clinical scoring (i.e. erythema, roughness, crevices), histopathological examination and eventually by checking the presence of the irritant chemical or its metabolite(s) in the blood or urine [15].

We have conducted several studies on barrier creams and/or gels [1], using both guinea pigs and humans. The principle of the experiments was to submit the skin to different irritant chemicals with and without the previous use of a protective cream or gel. The application of the irritant was short (15–60 min, depending on the nature of the irritant). Each experiment could therefore be considered as an acute exposure to a well-defined irritant, very often at a high concentration; this type of investigation was very demanding as regards barrier

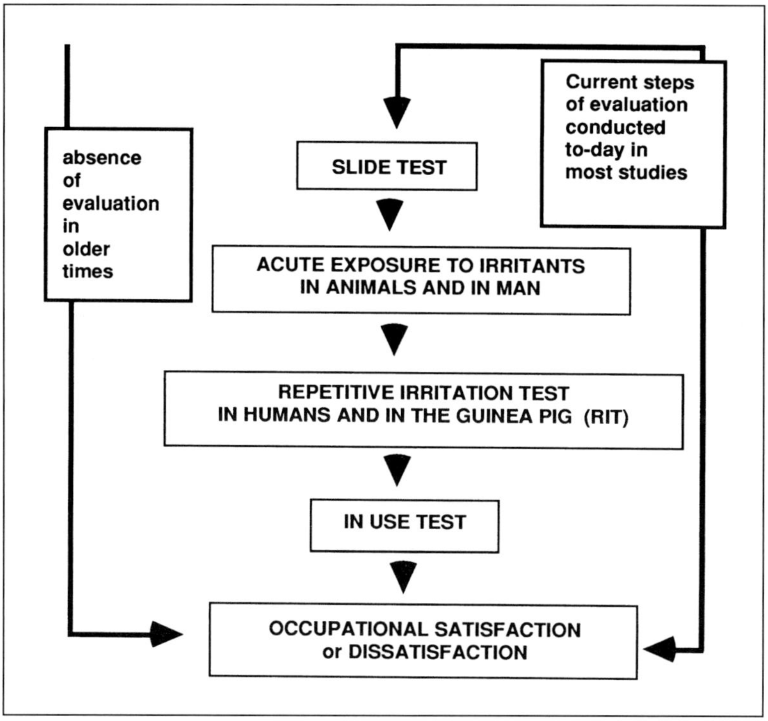

Fig. 1. Various steps of evaluation of the efficacy of barrier creams or gels.

qualities of the protective creams and on the other hand designed in such a manner that it was far away from the 'real' work condition at the work-place. Nevertheless, the advantages of the methodology were obvious because several types of investigations could be conducted simultaneoulsy: (a) evaluation of the skin morphological alterations by histopathological assessment; (b) evaluation of the skin functional status by non-invasive methods such as transepidermal water loss, Laser Doppler velocimetry, and skin capacitance; (c) biologial monitoring of organic solvents (such as n-hexane) in the blood.

In order to 'stick' more closely to the reality, Frosch et al. [17–21] developed two test models: the Repetitive Irritant Test (RIT) in guinea pigs and the RIT in humans (table 1), with a set of four standard irritants: 10% sodium laurylsulfate, 1% sodium hydroxide, 30% lactic acid and pure toluene. Hallmarks of both tests are the use of low, subtoxic doses of irritants, short-term repetitive application for 2 weeks (30 min, 9 applications), and quantification of the cutaneous irritant reaction by modern biophysical instruments such as

Table 1. RIT in humans

Healthy volunteers, back skin
Irritants at low subtoxic concentrations
Application daily for 30 min for 2 weeks with large Finn Chambers (total of 9 applications)
Skin protective cream (SPC) applied 30 min before the irritant
Control: Field without SPC on the same subject
Quantification of the skin reaction before exposure, on days 5 and 12
Erythema score (0–5)
TEWL
BFV

transepidermal water loss (TEWL) by evaporimetry, skin blood flow volume (BFV), by the Periflux Laser Doppler, stratum corneum hydration by skin capacitance or corneometry, and scoring of erythema on a 5+ scale.

Other tests are under evaluation nowadays, still closer to the realities of daily work, considering either industrial or nonindustrial exposure to irritant chemicals.

We have recently developed a new device using a circulation pump and therefore allowing a prolonged contact of skin with detergents in an open way, i.e. avoiding occlusion inherent to patch test procedures (repetitive open irritation test or ROIT). Many companies are conducting use tests, like for instance the hand or forearm wash procedure.

Assessment of Efficacy Limitations of Barrier Creams and Gels: An Overview

Skin protection against organic solvents by barrier creams or gels is limited. Some solvents, like trichlorethylene, toluene or xylene, penetrate easily into the skin through the protective creams or gels [13, 14]. Two French antisolvent gels, very similar in their formulation (mixture of proteins and lipoproteins, cellulose esters, triethanolamine, ethanol and water; pH 7.7), Antixol® (Laphi) and Phyprol 12® (Sorifa) have a real but incomplete effect on skin irritation due to n-hexane or acetone [12, 13], but this remains a controversial issue [17–21].

An antisolvent cream has been developed (Travabon®, Stockhausen), the formulation of which is as follows: water, talc pareth, glycerin, bentonite, sodium cocoyl isethionate, silica, PEG-75, sodium phosphate, titanium dioxide, algin (listed according to the CFTA nomenclature). We could demonstrate [22] that this formulation is efficacious – within certain limits – to prevent skin irritation provoked by n-hexane and – to a lesser extent – by toluene.

In short, it can be said that heavy exposure of skin to organic solvents leads to epidermal and dermal lesions that cannot be prevented by the use of barrier creams or gels; therefore, it requires protection by correctly designed gloves [23]. On the other hand, working intermittently with weakly irritant organic solvents in industry could benefit from the use of adapted barrier creams or gels [22].

In daily life, the risk of skin irritation due to direct contact with irritant chemicals dissolved in water is far more frequent and therefore deserves special attention. Common irritants include acids and alkalis, soaps, detergents, tensioactive agents, antiseptics, preservatives, amines, etc.

The need for effective barrier creams or gels is of prime importance. Unfortunately, 'ideal' protective products do not exist, but many formulations can be helpful in reducing skin irritation to an acceptable level.

Some dogmas can be reevaluated. For instance, silicones are of minor interest. It has been demonstrated that a 5% silicone cream (Anthydro®, Sorifa) was not significantly superior to its vehicle (i.e. the same cream without silicone) in preventing skin irritation due to a 10% sodium laurylsulfate solution [24] or to a 2% sodium hydroxide solution [25]. The old myth of silicone 'barrier' efficacy is therefore overestimated as far as current formulations of silicones are concerned. This observation is crucial, since silicone-based creams were banished in many plants due to the fact that adherence of paints or varnishes to metallic or plastic surfaces is impaired by silicones.

Another tenet can be thrown over without restraint: it was classical to admit that water in oil (W/O) emulsions (W/O creams, ointments) were designed to protect against irritants dissolved in water, whereas oil in water (O/W) emulsions (O/W creams, milks) were primarily effective against organic solvents.

Nowadays, this statement is no longer dogmatic due to the development of new galenic formulations [4].

Frosch et al. [17–21] have extensively studied the protective effect of several creams or gels available on the German market. The protection varies widely when various irritants are used: as an example Petrogard® (Salbe, Beiersdorf) is quite efficacious against sodium hydroxide, but offers a poor protection against lactic acid.

It is also very important to stress that foam gels, marketed as 'invisible gloves' such as Marly Skin® are of negligible interest against most irritants, either dissolved in water or in oil [3, 20].

It remains true that workers' satisfaction for using some barrier creams or gels is linked mainly to easier washing of the hands after work, which of course is cosmetically acceptable, providing that the cream or the gel has no harmful effect such as enhancing penetration of toxic substances through the skin. This last consideration enables us to remind all persons involved in a safety program that prevention measures must be carefully analyzed; the pros and the cons concerning the use of barrier creams of gels have to be closely weighed up.

Irritant and/or Allergenic Properties of Barrier Creams or Gels: Practical Implications

As mentioned above, protective creams or gels have to be applied on intact skin. In other words, they are not intended to be used on diseased skin, due to some irritant properties of many formulations [26, 27]. Apart from irritancy, they can also induce allergic contact dermatitis, mainly related to preservatives or fragrances [3]. Propyleneglycol, *p*-chlorometaxylenol, parabens and 2-bromo-2-nitropropane-1,3 diol (Bronopol®) are classic examples of provoking such allergies.

It is therefore of considerable importance that all components of the formula are known; ideally, complete labelling of the ingredients should be mentioned on the packages. In a skin-care program related to secondary prevention, it is for example recommended that workers suffering from hand eczema are routinely patch tested and, hence, given only supposedly well-tolerated creams or gels. Ingredients that give a positive patch test result should be systematically avoided.

In this respect, a close cooperation between occupational physicians, safety officers and dermatoallergologists is strongly advocated on a regular basis.

In our department we have reviewed 500 consecutive records of workers suffering from hand dermatitis. Sixteen of them had positive patch tests to preservatives, the current relevance of which was highly probable, related to the daily use of a barrier cream [unpubl. data].

Advent of Moisturizers for a Better Protection of the Skin against Irritants: Concept of Restoration versus Concept of Shielding

The use of protective ('barrier') creams or gels has so far been based upon the concept of 'shielding' the skin. The current formulations are supposed to contain repellent, complexing or film-forming ingredients into a cream or a gel base with good spreading properties, shear- and wash-off resistance and suited for use under daily working conditions. From the preceding paragraphs, it appears clearly that none of the available formulations meet all these criteria. The combination of all desired properties and the consumer demand for acceptable preparations is still a major challenge to the formulator [4].

A new approach to the problem of skin protection is no longer designed to 'shield' the skin with a barrier preparation but, on the contrary, is based on the concept of restoring the structure and/or function of the epidermal horny layer, damaged by various types of irritant chemicals.

This concept is derived from a better knowledge of the structural organization of the horny layer, primarily regulated by the lamellarly arranged lipid bilayers between the corneocytes. The barrier in the horny layer consists of ceramides and other skin lipids together with keratin. They form a so-called brick and mortar system in which the lipids form the mortar [28]. The epidermal lipids are mainly composed of ceramides, cholesterol and free fatty acids in approximatively equal quantities, originating from polar lipid precursors provided by the cells of the granular layer via the exocytosis of lamellar bodies contents. This now-growing understanding for the role, composition and architecture of the intercellular lipid bilayer structures is of fundamental importance to the formulator to design effective barrier restorative preparations aiming to supply the missing elements in the bilayer structure of epidermis. This approach could lead to re-establishment of the proper liquid crystalline structures to restore the water balance in the skin at the intercorneocyte level [29]. Such preparations should include the missing basic components of the intracellular lipid substance in a matrix which will enable the formation of the physiologically correct physical structures. In this perspective, it is noteworthy that there is a striking analogy between the organization of the lipid bilayers in the intercellular compartment of the horny layer and the structures achieved in mixtures of oil, water and emulsifying agents usually present in topical preparations [4]. For the time being, the composition of an ideal moisturizer is still under evaluation [28]. Furthermore, the idea of mixing ingredients in this type of formulation is progressing in many laboratories of cosmetic research. The transport of the various 'missing components (or ingredients)', through the superficial skin layers by diffusion will require conditions that cannot be optimal for all these components at the same time. It is urgently needed that new advanced formulation techniques are designed to deliver the proper ingredients at the right place.

We have shown recently in man [30] that the use of a moisturizing greasy cream (Excipial f.c.®), which is a W/O emulsion, has a good protective effect against moderate surfactant-induced irritation. The model used was very similar to that introduced by Frosch et al. [17], i.e. the RIT (see above). The surfactants were sodium laurylsulfate (2% in water) or sodium laurylethersulfate (10% in water). This protective effect was measured on human volunteers by the use of different noninvasive techniques, such as TEWL, skin capacitance and skin color reflectance. The most striking observations were: (a) the moisturizing cream Excipial f.c. was superior to conventional silicone or nonsilicone barrier creams, when used before applying the laurylethersulfate solution; (b) using Excipial f.c. before and after application of the surfactant provided a much higher degree of protection; this indicates that the 'restoration' of the skin barrier (horny layer) could be one of the best trails of research in the field of skin protection against irritants.

Another classic question is: Are cosmetic liposomes able to improve the skin barrier properties? A recent research [31] brings some answers to this question. It can be summarized as follows: liposomes do not pass through human stratum corneum intactly; liposome constituents as phospholipids interact with the skin lipids; the strength of interaction depends on the state of the liposomes (liquid state or gel state); liposome constituents penetrate the stratum corneum in a molecularly dispersed manner and may act as penetration enhancers; skin lipid interactions with liposome constituents result rather in reduction of the skin barrier function than in repair; observed skin hydration by topical application of liposomal preparations may be mainly caused by the occlusion effect of the vesicles.

Finally, the investigations performed with various human skin recombinants demonstrate that all systems developed so far approach the in vivo situation to a high extent. However, all recombinants still show signs of hyperproliferation, impaired barrier function and exhibit limited life span. The presence of the stratum corneum even with defective barrier function makes the human skin recombinants more useful for toxicity screening of topical products than the use of monocultures, since products can be applied in formulations and at concentrations used in daily life [32].

A further step could be the study of the protective effect of different formulations against irritants affecting the structure and function of the horny layer in this in vitro model [33].

It is concluded that in the design of new cosmetically acceptable formulations as an armentarium to the dermatologist, the challenges for the pharmaceutical formulator are significant and different for protective and restorative formulation products [34].

Conclusions

(1) 'Passive' protective creams and/or gels display unquestionable skin protective activities, within certain limits. Their efficacy depends on several factors, such as formulation of the cream, nature of the irritants and practical conditions at work. Much progress has still to be achieved.

(2) Silicones are of poor interest. It is possible that the use of new silicones providing a better physicochemical 'lattice' will modify our current view.

(3) 'Active' creams seem to be at a revival stage. Recent publications are promising in this direction.

(4) Moisturizers are gaining a lot of interest nowadays in skin protection. The mode of action is not based upon shielding the skin. They are claimed to offer a restoration of the horny layer of epidermis.

References

1 Mahmoud G, Lachapelle JM: Uses of a guinea pig model to evaluate the protective value of barrier creams and/or gels. Models Dermatol 1987;3:112–120.

2 Lachapelle JM: Principles of prevention and protection in contact dermatitis (with special reference to occupational dermatology); in Rycroft RJG, Menné T, Frosch PJ (eds): Textbook of Contact Dermatitis, ed 2. Berlin, Springer, 1995, pp 695–702.

3 Lachapelle JM, Frimat P, Tennstedt D, Ducombs G: Dermatologie professionnelle et de l'environnement. Paris, Masson, 1992, pp 1–400.

4 Korstanje C: Skin barrier creams: Concepts and properties of formulations. Clinical management of skin barrier problems. Yamanouchi Satellite Symposium 4th EADV Congress Brussels, October 13, 1995, pp 23–26.

5 Romaguera C, Grimalt F, Vilaplana J, et al: Formulation of a barrier cream against chromate. Contact Dermatitis, 1985;12:49–52.

6 Gawkrodger DJ, Healy J, Howe AM: The prevention of nickel contact dermatitis: A review of the use of binding agents and barrier creams. Contact Dermatitis 1995;32:257–265.

7 Fullerton A, Menné T: In vitro and in vivo evaluation of the effect of barrier gels in nickel contact allergy. Contact Dermatitis 1995;32:100–106.

8 Menné T: Prevention of nickel dermatitis. Allergologie 1995;18:447.

9 Grevelinck SA, Murrell DF, Olsen EA: Effectiveness of various barrier preparations in preventing and/or ameliorating experimentally produced Toxicodendron dermatitis. J Am Acad Dermatol 1992; 27:182–188.

10 Marks JG, Fowler JF, Sherertz E, Rietschel RL: Prevention of poison ivy/oak allergic contact dermatitis by quaternium-18 bentonite. Allergologie 1995;18:452.

11 Suskind RR: The present status of silicone protective creams. Indust Med Surg 1955;24: 413–416.

12 Mahmoud G, Lachapelle JM: Etude de l'efficacité d'un gel de protection anti-solvants, vis-à-vis de l'irritation cutanée provoquée par le n-hexane. Arch Mal Prof Méd Trav 1984;45:233–237.

13 Mahmoud G, Lachapelle JM: Evaluation expérimentale de l'efficacité de crèmes-barrière et de gels antisolvants dans la prévention de l'irritation cutanée provoquée par des solvants organiques. Cah Méd Trav 1985;22:163–168.

14 Mahmoud G, Lachapelle JM: Evaluation of the protective value of an antisolvent gel by laser Doppler flowmetry and histology. Contact Dermatitis 1985;13:14–19.

15 Lauwerys RR, Dath T, Lachapelle JM, Buchet JP, Roels H: The influence of two barrier creams on the percutaneous absorption of m-xylene in man. J Occup Med 1978;20:17–20.
16 Boman A, Wahlberg JE, Johanson G: A method for the study of the effect of barrier creams and protective gloves on the percutaneous absorption of solvents. Dermatologica 1982;164:157–160.
17 Frosch PJ, Schulze-Dirks A, Hoffmann M, et al: Efficacy of skin barrier creams. I. The repetitive irritation test (RIT) in the guinea pig. Contact Dermatitis 1993;28:94–100.
18 Frosch PJ, Schulze-Dirks A, Hoffmann M, et al: Efficacy of skin barrier creams. II. Ineffectiveness of a popular 'skin protector' against various irritants in the repetitive irritation test in the guinea pig. Contact Dermatitis 1993;29:74–77.
19 Frosch PJ, Kurte A, Pilz B: Efficacy of skin barrier creams. III. The repetitive irriation test (RIT) in humans. Contact Dermatitis 1993;29:113–118.
20 Frosch PJ, Kurte A: Efficacy of skin barrier creams. IV. The repetitive irritation test (RIT) with a set of 4 standard irritants. Contact Dermatitis 1994;31:161–168.
21 Frosch PJ, Pilz B: Hautschutz für Friseure – die Wirksamheit von 2 Hautschutzprodukten gegenüber Detergentien im Repetitiven Irritationstest. Dermatosen 1994;42:199–202.
22 Lachapelle JM, Nouaigui H, Marot L: Experimental study of the effects of a new protective cream against skin irritation provoked by the organic solvents n-hexane, trichlorethylene and toluene. Dermatosen 1990;38:19–23.
23 Mellström GA, Wahlberg JE, Maibach HI: Protective Gloves for Occupational Use. Boca Raton CRC Press, 1994, pp 1–314.
24 Nouaigui H, Antoine JL, Masmoudi ML, van Neste D, Lachapelle JM: Invasive and non-invasive studies of the protective effect of a silicone-containing cream and its vehicle on cutaneous irritation induced by sodium laurylsulphate. Ann Dermatol Venereol 1989;116:389–398.
25 Nouaigui H, Antoine JL, Lachapelle JM: An experimental study of the protective value of a silicone cream versus its vehicle against skin irritation provoked by sodium hydroxide. Arch Mal Prof 1988; 49:383–387.
26 Hogan DJ: The prognosis of hand eczema; in Menné T, Maibach HI (eds): Hand Eczema. Boca Raton, CRC Press. 1993, chap 27, pp 285–292.
27 Fowler JF Jr: Treatment of occupational dermatitis; in Hogan DJ (ed): Occupational Skin Disorders. New York, Igaka-Shoin, 1994, chap 9, pp 104–111.
28 Hannuksela M: Moisturizers in the prevention of contact dermatitis. Allergologie 1995;18:453.
29 Froebe CL, et al: Prevention of stratum corneum lipid phase transition in vitro by glycerol: An alternative mechanism for skin moisturization. J Soc Cosmet Chem 1990;41:51–65.
30 Perrenoud D, Lachapelle JM: Comparative study on 3 barrier creams and a fat-rich moisturizing cream. Allergologie 1994;3:110.
31 Junginger HE: Are cosmetic liposomes able to improve the skin barrier properties? J Appl Cosmetol 1995;13:120.
32 Ponec M: The use of in vitro skin recombinants to evaluate skin toxicity; in Rougier A, Goldberg AM, Maibach HI (eds): In vitro Skin Toxicology: Irritation, Phototoxicity, Sensitization. New York, Mary Ann Liebert, 1994, pp 107–116.
33 Fartasch M: Human barrier formation and reaction to irritation. Curr Probl Dermatol. Basel, Karger, 1995, vol 23, pp 95–103.
34 Lachapelle JM: The efficacy of protective creams. Allergologie 1995;18:452.

J.M. Lachapelle, Unit of Dermato-Allergology and Dermato-Immunology,
Laboratory of Occupational and Environmental Dermatology, Catholic University of Louvain,
30, Clos Chapelle-aux-Champs UCL 3033, B–1200 Brussels (Belgium)

Elsner P, Lachapelle JM, Wahlberg JE, Maibach HI (eds): Prevention of Contact Dermatitis. Curr Probl Dermatol. Basel, Karger, 1996, vol 25, pp 193–205

Percutaneous Penetration (Dermatopharmacokinetics) in Evaluating Barrier Creams

Hongbo Zhai, Howard I. Maibach

Department of Dermatology, School of Medicine, University of California, San Francisco, Calif., USA

Barrier creams (BC) are designed to prevent or reduce the penetration of harmful agents into skin, preventing skin lesions and/or other toxic effects from dermal exposure.

Different in vivo and in vitro methods have been used to evaluate their efficacy. Pharmacokinetic studies provide kinetic details and mechanistic insights that have the potential to supplement traditional clinical studies.

This chapter summarizes the methodology to quantify percutaneous absorption in the evaluation of the efficacy of barrier creams and summarizes the results of such penetration studies.

Pharmacokinetic versus Pharmacodynamic

Pharmacokinetics deals with the relationship between drug concentration in the body and the rate and amount of drug presented to the body. Pharmacodynamics deals with the drug effect. Pharmacokinetic (PK) models describe drug concentrations as a function of dose and time. Pharmacodynamic (PD) models describe the relationship between the concentration at the effect site and the effect [1].

Pharmacokinetic methods may nonetheless be useful in the determination of bioequivalence of topical dermatological products [2, 3]. These methods can generally be divided into attempts to assess rate and extent of drug absorption locally (dermatopharmacokinetics) and more standard methods to assess rate and extent of drug absorption at the site of application by measure of systemic concentration of the drug or its metabolites [4]. Wester and Maibach [5] described percutaneous absorption in terms of ten steps with examples of bioavailability. Most of the preceding discussion of pharmacokinetics focuses on bioavailability from a percutaneous route of administration. Bioavailability can be defined as the rate and extent to which the administered drug ingredient or therapeutic moiety is absorbed from a drug formulation and becomes available at the site of drug action and/or reaches the general circulation. Other pharmacokinetic parameters are the distribution, metabolism, and excretion of the applied chemical [6]. We focus here on the penetration of chemicals concerning the effects of barrier cream. However, the effect of barrier creams may depend on the total pharmacokinetics of the chemical.

Pharmacokinetics: Advantages

One advantage of dermal pharmacokinetic models over traditional in vivo methods is the ability to accurately describe nonlinear biochemical and physical processes. Describing skin penetration based on blood concentrations or excretion rates as 'percent absorbed' assumes all processes have a simple linear relationship with the exposure concentration. When nonlinear processes occur in the absorption, distribution, metabolism, or elimination of a chemical, describing absorption as 'percent absorbed' may be misleading. Dermal absorption may not be linear when there is binding or metabolism in the skin or when skin blood flow is a limiting factor. Many biochemical processes in the body are nonlinear. A quantitative description of saturable kinetics in the model may allow it to be predictive of blood or tissue concentrations from various doses. Another would be to estimate the rate of skin metabolism in the skin. Proper comparison of the metabolite production after application to the skin at several concentrations allows the metabolic parameters in the skin to be estimated [7].

Quantifying Penetration: Method

In studying percutaneous absorption, a detection method is needed to detect the penetration. The analysis can be performed by measuring radioactivity using a labeled compound or a chemical assay. The biologic response is dynamic. Assay of compound is usually done following penetration directly into a collection vessel (in vitro) or indirectly in biologic fluids or tissues (in vivo).

The in vitro technique entails placing excised skin in a diffusion chamber, applying compound to its surface, and then assaying for compound in the collection vessel on the other side. Excised human and animal skin are used, and the skin may be wholly intact or separated into epidermis or dermis. Artificial membranes have also been used. A major advantage of in vitro systems is that they allow for absorption measurements through skin of chemicals too toxic to test in human subjects. Absorption rates and skin metabolism can be measured in the in vitro system because sampling is performed directly beneath the barrier layer. Skin metabolism can be studied in viable skin without interference from systemic metabolic processes. Finally, absorption measurements are obtained much more easily from diffusion cells than from analysis of biological specimens from clinical studies. Other advantages of the in vitro technique are that the method is easy to use and the results are obtained quickly. A disadvantage is that the collection bath is saline, which is compatible with hydrophilic compounds but not with hydrophobic compounds. In vivo the penetrating compound does not pass completely through the dermis but is removed by capillaries in the dermis.

Percutaneous absorption in vivo is usually determined by the indirect method of measuring radioactivity in excreta following topical application of the compound. Plasma levels of compounds are often low following topical application, usually below the assay detection level. The compound, often labelled, is applied to the skin and the total amount of radioactivity excreted in urine or urine plus feces is then determined. The amount of radioactivity retained in the body or excreted by some route not assayed (CO_2) is corrected for by determining the amount of radioactivity excreted following parental administration. Feldmann and Maibach [8–10] developed a protocol for measurement of percutaneous absorption in man. This method involves quantifying absorption on the basis of the percent of radioactivity excreted in urine following application of a known amount of the labeled compound to the skin.

Pharmacokinetic Data

Lachapelle's group [11–14] utilized a guinea pig model to evaluate the protective value of barrier creams and/or gels by laser doppler flowmetry and histological assessment. In addition, the blood concentration of n-hexane of the control group and the gel-pretreated group was determined. Figure 1 shows the partial results [14]. It was possible to correlate results obtained by invasive (blood levels) and noninvasive techniques.

Earlier, Sadler et al. [15] performed qualitative tests to evaluate the efficiency of barrier creams. One method used the fluorescence of a dyestuff and

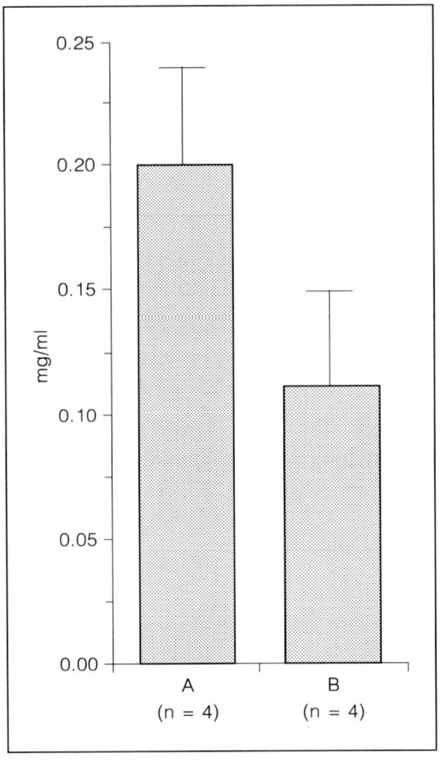

Fig. 1. Mean ± SD (μg/ml) of blood levels of n-hexane in two groups of guinea pigs exposed for 30 min. A = Control group; B = gel-pretreated group ($p < 0.05$). From Mahmoud and Lachapelle [14], with modification.

eosin as an indicator to measure penetration and the rates of penetration of water through barrier creams; this is rapid and simple, but provides only a rough quantitative estimate. They introduced an apparatus for measuring the permeability of films of barrier creams.

Wahlberg [16, 17] employed an isotope technique disappearance measurement for studying the inhibiting effect of barrier cream on chromate (^{51}Cr) percutaneous absorption in guinea pigs. Data are presented in table 1 and in figure 2 [17]. In this series 2,4 (Indulona®) and 6–10 (Ivosin®) absorption decreased as a result of pretreatment. In some cases the disappearance technique was not sufficiently sensitive to permit quantitative determination. The method, disappearance measurements [18], permitted a differentiation between barrier creams of different types, volumes per unit area and intervals between application of cream and chromate.

Langford [19] introduced in vitro studies conducted to determine the efficacy of the formulated FC-resin complex included solvent penetration through treated filter paper, solvent repellency on treated pigskin, and penetra-

Table 1. Influence of Indulona and Ivosin on the percutaneous absorption of 0.017 *M* chromate solution $K \times 10^5\ min^{-1}$. From [17], with modification

Series No.	Barrier cream	Volume applied ml/cm^2	Interval[1] min	<3.4	3.4–6.6	6.7–10.1	10.2–13.5	>13.6	Mean relative absorption $K \times 10^5\ min^{-1}$ 10 exp.	χ^2 (c), analysis of variance (v) compared with series 1
				n	n	n	n	n		
1	no barrier cream			–	4	4	–	2	8.8 ± 1.4^2	–
2	Indulona	0.05	1	3	2	4	–	1	$(5.7–6.7)^3$	$0.05 < p < 0.10$ (c)
3	Indulona	0.10	1	–	3	4	1	2	9.0 ± 1.2^2	$p > 0.2$ (v)
4	Indulona	0.10	15	4	1	3	2	–	$(5.5–6.8)^3$	$0.02 < p < 0.05$ (c)
5	Indulona	0.15	1	–	5	–	5	–	8.2 ± 0.1^2	$p > 0.2$ (v)
6	Ivosin	0.025	1	2	2	3	3	–	$(6.7–7.3)^3$	$0.10 < p < 0.20$ (c)
7	Ivosin	0.05	1	7	1	2	–	–	$(2.1–4.5)^3$	$0.001 < p < 0.01$ (c)
8	Ivosin	0.10	1	8	–	2	–	–	$(1.8–4.5)^3$	$p < 0.001$ (c)
9	Ivosin	0.10	15	5	5	–	–	–	$(2.5–4.2)^3$	$0.001 < p < 0.01$ (c)
10	Ivosin	0.15	1	5	3	2	–	–	$(3.2–4.7)^3$	$0.001 < p < 0.01$ (c)

[1] Interval between application of barrier cream and test substance.
[2] Standard error.
[3] See text.

tion of radio-tagged sodium lauryl-sulfate through treated hairless mouse skin. The penetration rate of radio-tagged sodium laurylsulfate/ETOH through hairless mouse skin is shown in figure 3.

Reiner et al. [20] examined the protective effect of ointments both on guinea pig skin in vitro and on guinea pigs in vivo. The permeation of 'Toxic agent 4'® through unprotected and protected skin within 10 h is plotted in figure 4 as a function of time. The permeation values were determined both radiologically and enzymatically. The permeation of the 'Toxic agent 4' was markedly reduced by both the polyethylene glycol ointment base and the ointments containing active substance. In in vivo experiments on guinea pigs mortality was greater after applying the toxic agent to unprotected skin. All formulations with nucleophilic substances markedly reduced the mortality rate.

Loden [21] evaluated the effect of 4 barrier creams on the absorption of (^3H)-water (^{14}C)-benzene and (^{14}C)-formaldehyde into excised human skin. The control and the barrier-cream-treated skins were exposed to the test substance for 0.5 h, whereupon the amount absorbed was determined. The results indi-

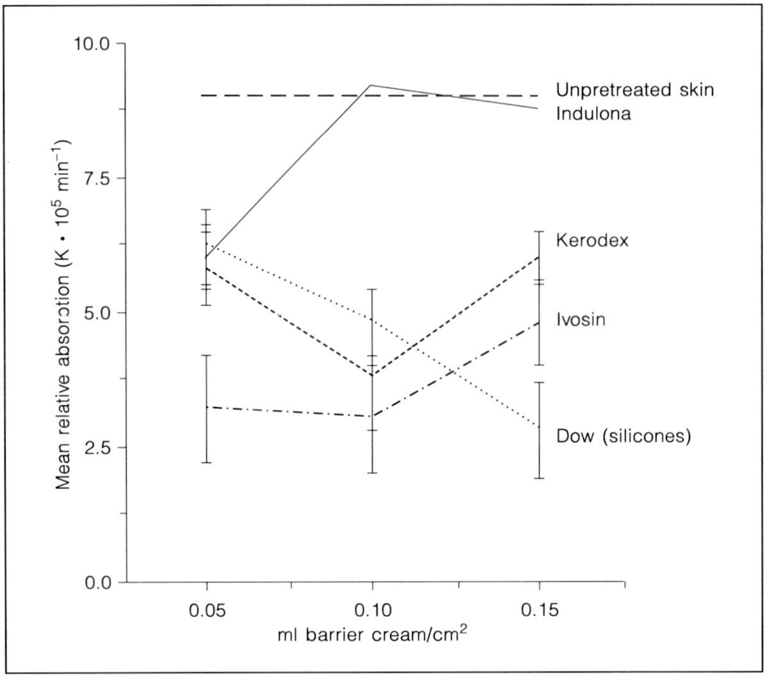

Fig. 2. The effect of four barrier creams on the percutaneous absorption of a 0.017 *M* aqueous solution of chromate. Three different volumes per unit area (ml/cm^2) were studied. From Wahlberg [17], with modification.

cated that the experimental cream 'water barrier' reduced the absorption of water and benzene but not formaldehyde. Kerodex 71® cream slightly reduced the absorption of benzene and formaldehyde. Petrogard® and 'Solvent barrier'® did not affect the absorption of any of the substances studied. The results are shown in figure 5. One of the main advantages of the method is the use of human skin. The effects of the barrier cream on both the skin and the test substance mimic the in vivo situation. Another advantage is that the method is not only qualitative, i.e. distinguishes between the creams, but also quantitative, i.e. a certain degree of alteration in absorption is obtained.

Treffel et al. [22] developed a method to measure in vitro on human skin the effectiveness of barrier creams against three dyes (eosin, methyl violet and oil red O) with different n-octanol/water partition coefficients (0.19, 29.8 and 165, respectively). Barrier creams were assayed by measurements of the dyes in the epidermis of protected skin samples after 30 min application. Penetration depths of the dyes into the stratum corneum are shown in figure 6.

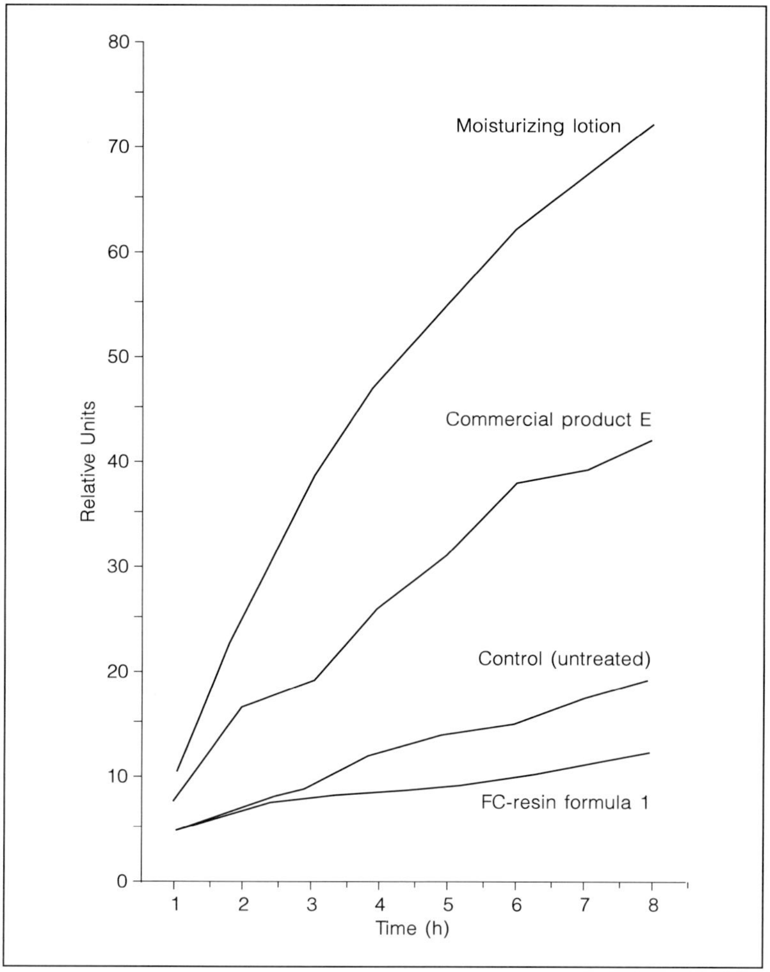

Fig. 3. Penetration rate of radio-tagged sodium laurylsulfate/ETOH through hairless mouse skin. From Langford [19], with modification.

The ΔTTC (%) related to the number of the cellophane tape strips made from the skin sample controls. The dyes were present in high amounts in the superficial layers of the stratum corneum; the Δ-TTC due to eosin in the first strip was lower than that obtained with both the other dyes but this was not statistically significant. The results show oil red O to penetrate in greater amounts into the deep layers of the stratum corneum. The amount of the three dyes at the bottom of the stratum corneum remains, however, low. The

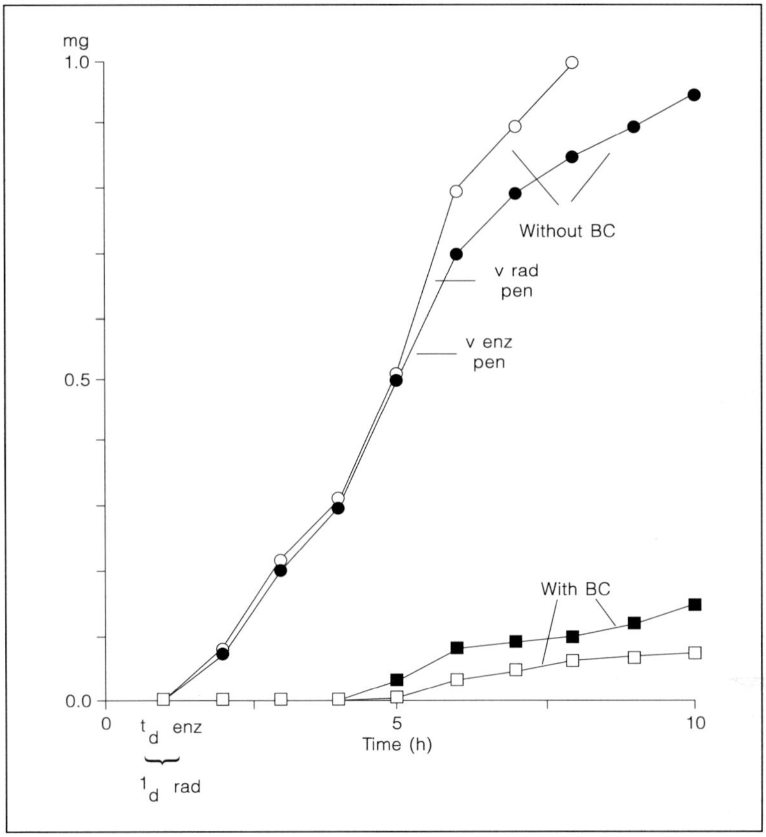

Fig. 4. Permeation of the toxic agent 4 through unprotected and protected skin as a function of time. o = Rad data; ● = enzyme data; BC = reactive PEG ointment such as S4-S8. From Reiner et al. [20], with modification.

efficacy of barrier creams against the three dyes shown in several cases disagree with the manufacturer's information. There was no correlation between the galenic parameters of the assayed products and the level of protection, indicating that neither the water content nor the consistency of the formulations influenced the protection effectiveness.

Fullerton and Menne [23] evaluated the protective effect of various ethylenediaminetetraacetate (EDTA) barrier gels against nickel contact allergy using in vitro and in vivo methods. About 30 mg of barrier gel was applied on the epidermal side of the skin in vitro. A nickel disc was applied above the gel. After 24 h of application, the nickel disc was removed from and the

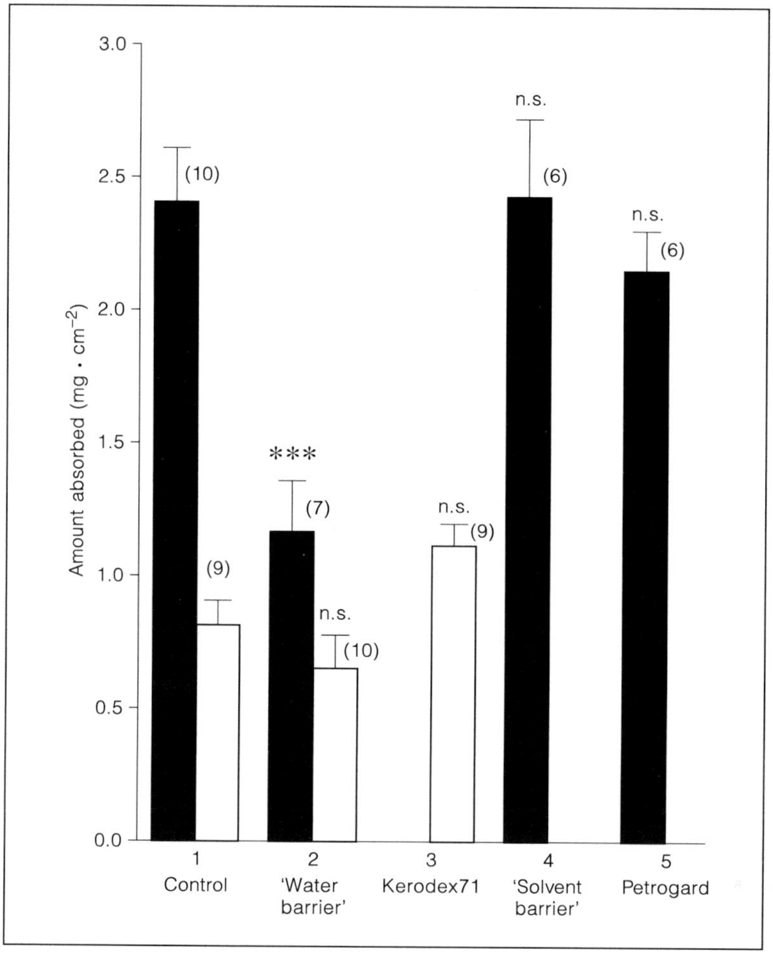

Fig. 5. The amount of water absorbed into control skin and skin treated with 4 different barrier creams during 0.5 h of exposure. Skin from 2 donors was used. Values are means ± SE of the number of experiments within parenthesis. *** $p<0.001$; n.s. = not significantly different from control. From Loden [21], with modification.

epidermis separated from the dermis. The nickel content in epidermis and dermis was quantified by absorption differential pulse voltammetry (ADPV). The distributions of nickel in epidermis and dermis after 24 h of occluded application of the 2 nickel discs made from alloy A and alloy B is seen in figure 7. They found that the amount of nickel in the epidermal skin layer

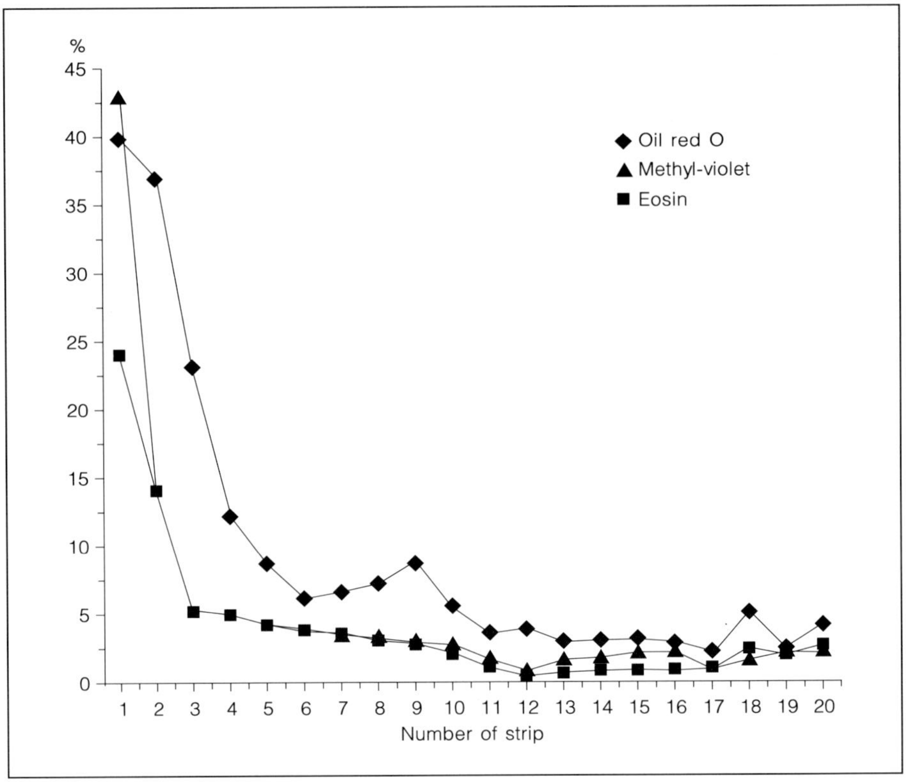

Fig. 6. Δ total color change measurement in the stratum corneum expressed in percentage. From Treffel et al. [22], with modification.

after application of the barrier gels was significantly reduced compared to the untreated control.

In vivo patch testing of nickel-sensitive patients was performed using nickel discs made of metal alloy A and using Carbopol barrier gel systems with and without added EDTA (gel type A and B). Test preparations and nickel discs were removed 1 day after applications and the test sites evaluated. The results of patch testing showed that reduction in positive test reactions was highly significant.

Wester et al. [24] utilized 1% concentration of [^{35}S]-sodium laurylsulfate (SLS) to measure the protective effective of Bentoquatam (Q18B) gel by human cadaver skin with diffusion system. The results are shown in figure 8. A combined paired t test for all formulations showed Q18B to significantly decrease sodium laurylsulfate skin absorption.

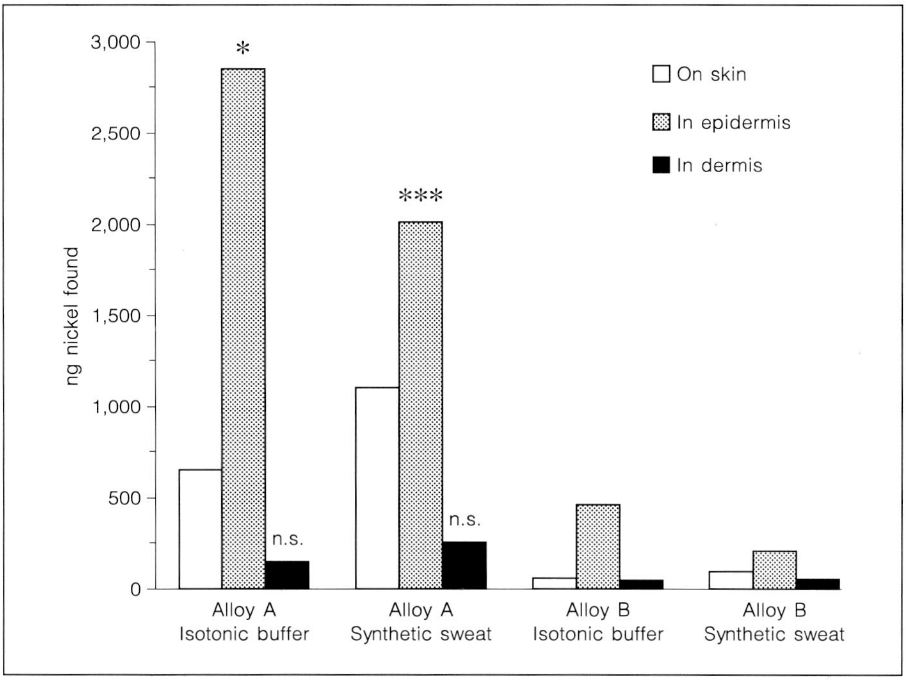

Fig. 7. Distribution of nickel in epidermis and dermis after 24 h occluded application of 2 nickel discs made from alloy A and alloy B. Recipient mediums were isotonic phosphate buffer and synthetic sweat (skin from donor A). Statistics: 2-sample t test comparing mean skin compartment distribution of nickel after application of alloy B and alloy A. Comparison for isotonic phosphate buffer and synthetic sweat as recipient medium, respectively. n.s. = No significance; * $p < 0.05$, *** $p < 0.001$. From Fullerton and Menne [23], with modification.

Conclusion

The choice of methods of measurement of the protective effect of barrier creams is guided by two main criteria: efficacy and safety. In vitro methods are recommended as a screening procedure for barrier cream candidates because of their simplicity and speed. Animals may be used to generate kinetic data. Percutaneous absorption in pigs and monkeys shows a closer similarity to that in humans. But no one animal, with its complex anatomy and biology, will simulate the penetration in humans for all compounds. Therefore, the best estimate of human percutaneous absorption is determined by in vivo studies in humans.

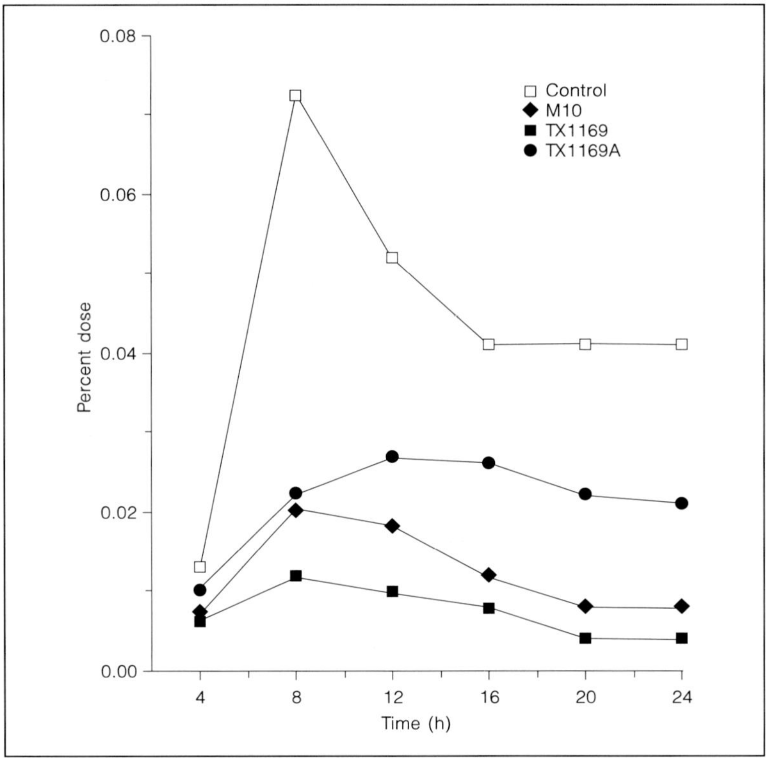

Fig. 8. Formulations for inhibitor of sodium laurylsulfate skin absorption. From Wester et al. [24], with modification.

The accuracy of measurements of the efficacy of barrier creams depends on the use of proper methodology. We believe that sensible, standardized and hopefully widely accepted methods are indicated. Pharmacokinetics should play one step in their development; the final arbiter will be the clinical information from well-controlled human assays.

References

1 Suneel K, Gupta E, Bashaw ED, Hwang SS: Pharmacokinetic and pharmacodynamic modeling of transdermal products; in Shah VP, Maibach HI (eds): Topical Drug Bioavailability, Bioequivalence, and Penetration. New York, Plenum Press, 1993, pp 311–332.

2 Shah VP, Flynn GL, Guy RH, Maibach HI, Schaefer H, Skelly JP, Weater RC, Yacobi A: In vivo percutaneous penetration/absorption. Pharm Res 1991;8:1071–1075.

3 Guy RH, Guy AH, Maibach HI, Shah VP: The bioavailability of dermatological and other topically administered drugs. Pharm Res 1986;3:253–262.

4 Shah VP, Hare D, Dighe SV, Williams RL: Bioequivalence of topical dermatological products; in Shah VP, Maibach HI (eds): Topical Drug Bioavailability, Bioequivalence, and Penetration. New York, Plenum Press, 1993, pp 393–413.
5 Wester RC, Maibach HI: Cutaneous pharmacokinetics: 10 steps to percutaneous absorption. Drug Metab Rev 1983;14:169–205.
6 Wester RC, Maibach HI: In vivo percutaneous absorption; in Marzulli FN, Maibach HI (eds): Dermatotoxicology, ed 4. New York, Hemisphere, 1991, pp 75–96.
7 McDougal JN: Physiologically based pharmacokinetic modeling; in Marzulli FN, Maibach HI (eds): Dermatotoxicology, ed 4. New York, Hemisphere, 1991, pp 37–60.
8 Feldmann RJ, Maibach HI: Percutaneous penetration of steroids in man. J Invest Derm 1969;52: 89–94.
9 Feldman RJ, Maibach HI: Absorption of some organic compounds through the skin in man. J Invest Derm 1970;54:339–404.
10 Feldmann RJ, Maibach HI: Percutaneous penetration of some pesticides and herbicides in man. Toxicol Appl Pharmacol 1974;28:126–132.
11 Mahmoud G, Lachapelle JM, Neste DV: Histological assessment of skin damage by irritants: Its possible use in the evaluation of a 'barrier cream'. Contact Dermatitis 1984;11:179–185.
12 Mahmoud G, Lachapelle JM: Evaluation of the protective value of an antisolvent gel by laser Doppler flowmetry and histology. Contact Dermatitis 1985;13:14–19.
13 Lachapelle JM, Nouaigui H, Marot L: Experimental study of the effects of a new protective cream against skin irritation provoked by the organic solvents n-hexane, trichlorethylene and toluene. Dermatosen Heft 1990;38:19–23.
14 Mahmoud G, Lachapelle JM: Uses of a guinea pig model to evaluate the protective value of barrier creams and/or gels; in Maibach HI, Lowe NJ (eds): Models in Dermatology, vol 4. Basel, Karger, 1987, pp 112–120.
15 Sadler CGA, Marriott RH: The evaluation of barrier creams. Br Med J 1946;23:769–773.
16 Wahlberg JE: Absorption-inhibiting effect of barrier creams. Berufs-Dermatosen 1971;19:197–207.
17 Wahlberg JE: Anti-chromium barrier creams. Dermatologica 1972;145:175–181.
18 Wahlberg JE: Disappearance measurements: A method for studying percutaneous absorption of isotope-labelled compounds emitting γ-rays. Acta Derm Venereol 1965;45:397–414.
19 Langford NP: Fluorochemical resin complexes for use in solvent repellent hand creams. Am Ind Hyg Assoc J 1978;39:33–40.
20 Reiner R, Rossmann K, Hooidonk CV, Ceulen BI, Bock J: Ointments for the protection against organophosphate poisoning. Arzneimittel-Forsch 1982;32:630–633.
21 Loden M: The effect of 4 barrier creams on the absorption of water, benzene, and formaldehyde into excised human skin. Contact Dermatitis 1986;14:292–296.
22 Treffel P, Gabard B, Juch R: Evaluation of barrier creams: An in vitro technique on human skin. Acta Derm Venereol 1994;74:7–11.
23 Fullerton A, Menne T: In vitro and in vivo evaluation of the effect of barrier gels in nickel contact allergy. Contact Dermatitis 1995;32:100–106.
24 Wester RC, Hartway T, Serranzana S, Zhai H, Maibach HI: In vitro percutaneous absorption of sodium lauryl sulfate (SLS) in human skin protected with Bentoquatam (Q-18B) gels. In preparation.

Prof. Howard I. Maibach, Department of Dermatology, University of California, School of Medicine, Box 0989, Surge 110, San Francisco, CA 94143–0989 (USA)

Elsner P, Lachapelle JM, Wahlberg JE, Maibach HI (eds): Prevention of Contact Dermatitis. Curr Probl Dermatol. Basel, Karger, 1996, vol 25, pp 206–213

Barrier Recompensation Mechanisms

A. M. Grunewald[a], *M. Gloor*[a], *P. Kleesz*[b]

[a] Dermatological Clinic of Karlsruhe Municipal Hospital (Director: Prof. Dr. *M. Gloor*), Karlsruhe, and
[b] Arbeitsmedizinischer Dienst der Berufsgenossenschaft Nahrungsmittel und Gaststätten (Director: Prof. Dr. Ing *S. Radandt* and *R. Grieshaber*), Mannheim, Germany

Washing of the skin with a surfactant leads to delipidation and dehydration of the stratum corneum, a pH shift of the skin into the alkaline region, a barrier function deterioration and in the case of an aggressive irritant to visible inflammatory changes like reddening and scaling of the skin [1]. The repetitive application of skin irritants leads to a further deterioration of skin functions compared to a single application of the same irritant. Nevertheless, the degree of deterioration after repetitive irritation is lower than to be expected with a cumulative irritation response [2]. In a previous study of our working group we clinically observed reddening and scaling on the second to fourth day of repetitive washings with 0.01 mol/l sodium laurylsulfate (SLS) as the irritant solution. Despite continuous washing, there was an improvement of clinical symptoms after 4–5 days [unpubl. data]. These clinical observations let assume a recompensation mechanism of the skin following repetitive irritation. In this study we want to evaluate a possible training effect of the skin using corneometry, transepidermal water loss (TEWL), laser doppler flow (LD) and pH-metry.

Material and Methods

Experimental Subjects

The investigations were carried out on 10 healthy subjects. The average age of the subjects was 25 years, ranging between 18 and 34 years, with 60% female and 40% male.

Irritant Solution

We used SLS (Texapon K12, Caesar & Loretz GmbH, Hilden, Germany) 0.01 mol/l as the surfactant.

Experimental Set-Up

Washings were performed on the right or the left forearm of each subject, while the other forearm was kept as control. Washing was done 50 × with a 250-gram foam rubber roller soaked 3 × in the wash solution [1]. This washing procedure was repeated 3 × /day under control in the laboratory.

Measurement Procedures

All measurements took place in a climatized room of our clinic. Room temperature was at 21 ± 1 °C and the relative humidity was 45 ± 5%. The subjects had to acclimatize to these conditions for 30 min before the experiment. To avoid interactions between the different bioengineering methods we decided to have 4 independent test areas on each forearm. Bioengineering methods were used in the following order.

(a) Corneometry (CM 820, Courage & Khazaka, Cologne, Germany): relative values were obtained. Eight measurements were carried out at closely spaced sites at a time and their mean was calculated [3].

(b) TEWL (TM 210. Courage & Khazaka): the measured signals were only recorded when a constant value had been detected for 30 s (variation allowed was <0.5 g/m^2 h) [4].

(c) LD (Pf2, Perimed, Sweden): relative values were obtained. Values were only recorded after a constant signal had been observed for at least 2 min [5].

(d) pH-metry (PH 900, Courage & Khazaka): measurements were carried out in a droplet of distilled water and expressed as the mean of three recordings [6].

Time Points of Measurement

Measurements were done before (day 0) and at day 1, 2, 3, 5, 8, 10 and 14 after the beginning of repetitive washing. The last wash had to be 12 h before each measurement. No cosmetic treatment of the forearms was allowed.

Statistical Assessment

Comparison of values were carried out between washed site and control of each day of measurement. Results are given as median values and the distribution is expressed as the lower (1st) and upper (3rd) quartiles. The Wilcoxon signed-ranked test was used. With a high number of statistical tests being performed false-positive significances at the 5% level may be expected. Nevertheless, multiple p values of <0.05 in one time course of one test series (i.e. 1st, 2nd, 3rd, 5th day measurements) confirm the correctness of the statistical assessment. Therefore, they were interpreted as a significant result. We postulated in hypothesis A that differences between the washed site and the control site (Δq) are not lower on day 0 compared to day 3, i.e. showing no deterioration of skin functions due to repetitive irritation, and in hypothesis B that Δq is not lower on day 14 than on day 3, i.e. there is no regeneration of the skin following day 3.

Results

See table 1 and 2 and figures 1–4 for detailed results. All four skin function parameters show a distinct deterioration after the beginning of repetitive washing with a maximum at day 1 (pH and corneometry), at day 3 (LD) or

Table 1. Results of the bioengineering method measurements: median values (1st/3rd quartiles in parentheses)

		Day 0	Day 1	Day 2	Day 3	Day 5	Day 8	Day 10	Day 14
Corneometry	washed	64(59/66)	47(43/53) *	52(48/56) *	54(50/58) *	55(50/60) *	57(49/62)	56(51/63)	59(54/63)
	control	64(61/67)	68(66/70)	67(59/70)	65(62/70)	68(69/70)	61(54/70)	62(56/65)	60(55/65)
TEWL	washed	2.9(2.6/3.2)	3.6(3.1/4.0) *	4.2(3.8/4.7) *	3.8(3.3/4.2) *	5.4(4.8/6.8) *	3.9(3.2/4.5) *	3.6(3.1/4.7) *	3.8(3.1/4.6) +
	control	2.6(2.2/3)	2.2(2/2.8)	2.7(2.6/3.4)	2(1.8/2.8)	3.2(2.8/3.5)	2.4(2.1/2.6)	2.5(2.3/3.1)	2.7(2.1/3.2)
LD	washed	12(10/13)	13.5(12/15)	15(13/17) +	16(15/18) +	16.5(14/18) *	14.5(14/18)	14(10/16)	11.5(10/17)
	control	10(9/14)	11.5(9/14)	13(8/14)	13.5(9/15)	12(10/14)	12.5(11/14)	12(10/14)	11.5(10/14)
pH-metry	washed	5.1(4.8/5.4)	6.3(6.1/6.5) *	5.4(5.1/6.2)	5.6(5.4/6.3) *	5.6(5.3/6.5)	5.7(5.3/6.0) +	5.6(4.8/5.7)	5.2(5.0/5.6)
	control	5(4.8/5.3)	5.1(4.9/5.4)	5(4.43/5.6)	5(4.5/5.2)	5.2(5/6.2)	5(4.5/5.4)	5(4.5/5.4)	5(4.5/5.4)

For significances see legend to figures 1–4.

Table 2. Comparison of the differences Δq (washed site minus control site values) on day 0, day 3 and day 14 for the different bioengineering methods used ($^{+}p < 0.05$; $^{*}p < 0.01$)

	Day 0		Day 3		Day 14
Corneometry	–0.25 (–1.9/0.2)	*	–11.35 (–13/–9.3)	*	–1.05 (–5/0)
TEWL	0.1 (0/0.7)	*	1.4 (1/1.9)		1.3 (0.8/1.6)
		* (day 0–day 14)			
LD	0 (–2/3)	+	3.5 (2.5)	+	0.5 (–1/3)
pH-metry	0.08 (0/0.2)	*	0.65 (0.2/1.03)	+	0.2 (0.2/0.36)

at day 5 (TEWL), respectively (fig. 1–4). Following the maximum of deterioration the measured corneometry, LD and pH values slowly decline and values are close to control values at day 14 again, despite continuous repetitive washings. Comparing the corneometry, LD and pH value differences Δq (washed site minus control site values), there are significant differences detectable between day 0 and day 3 concerning all bioengineering methods tested as well as between day 3 and day 14 concerning corneometry, LD and pH, in contrary to our hypothesis. No significant differences are detectable between day 0 and day 14. Our hypothesis A therefore has to be dismissed, i.e. repetitive washing leads to a deterioration of skin function. Hypothesis B has to be dismissed concerning corneometry, LD and pH, i.e. a continuation of repetitive washing beyond day 3 leads to regeneration of the skin. Concerning barrier function there is recompensation following day 5 leading to a steady state of TEWL values despite a continuation of repetitive washing. Nevertheless, there is no significant regeneration of TEWL values until day 14.

Discussion

Following repetitive subclinical irritation by a surfactant there is a cumulative response during the first days of irritation. This result is comparable with the results of earlier investigations of our own as well as other working groups [2, 7]. In 1981, Malten [8] postulated the mechanisms of barrier damage

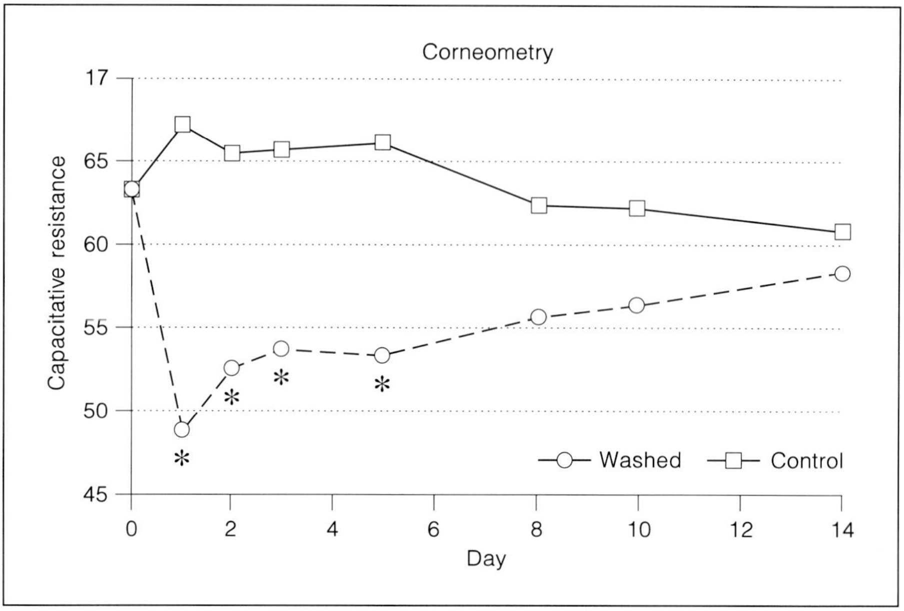
Corneometry
Capacitative resistance
17
65
60
55
50
45
0
2
4
6
8
10
12
14
Day
Washed
Control

1

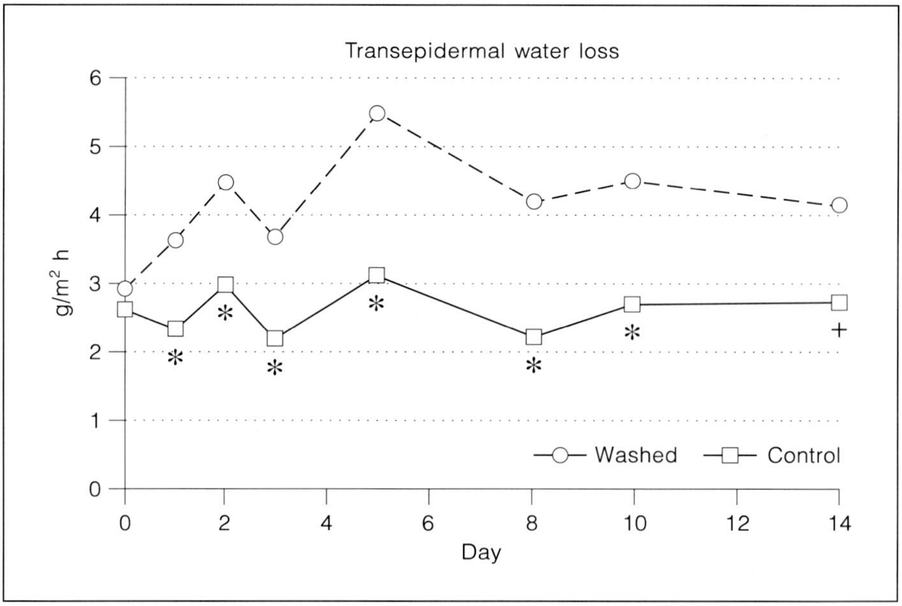
Transepidermal water loss
g/m² h
6
5
4
3
2
1
0
0
2
4
6
8
10
12
14
Day
Washed
Control

2

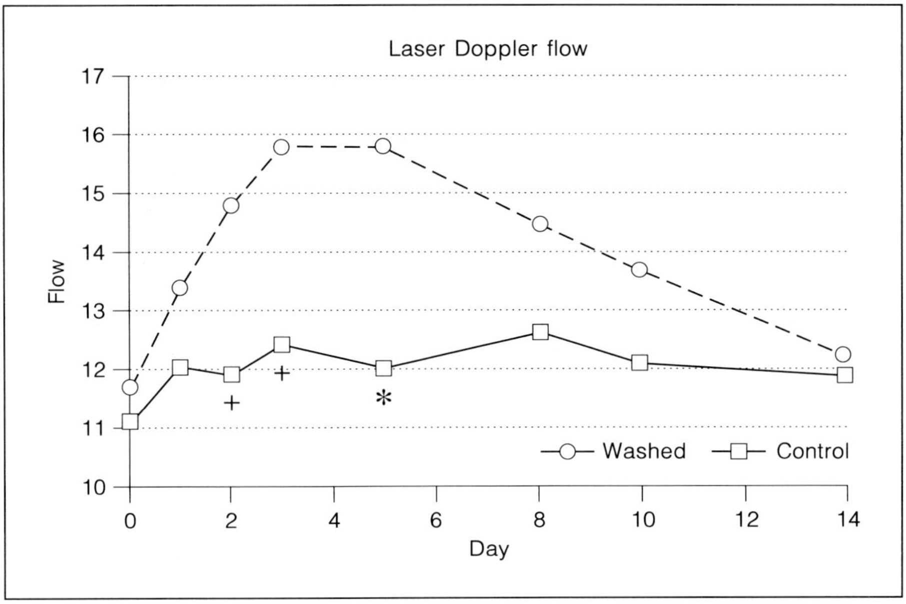

3

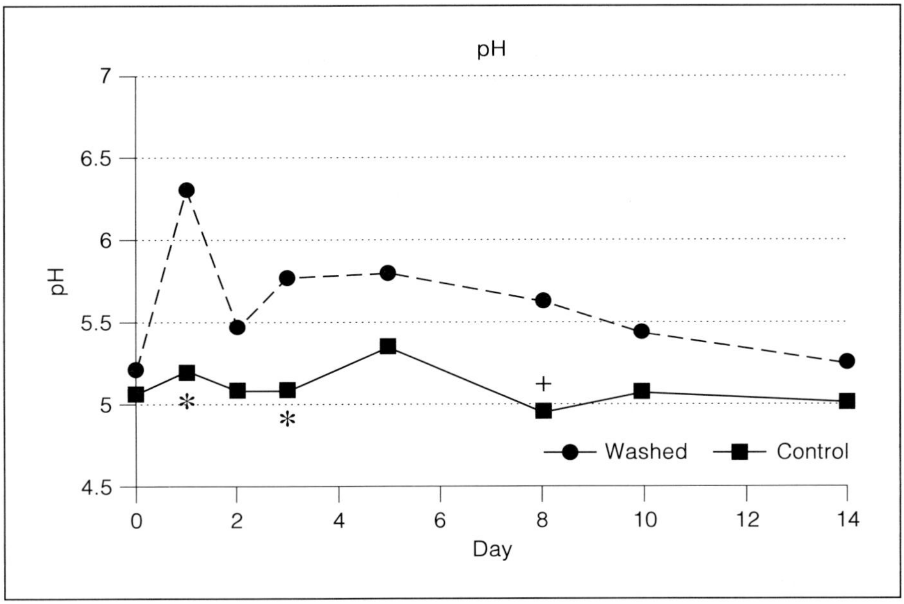

4

Fig. 1–4. Mean values of the bioengineering method measurements on the washed site and the control site. For detailed results, see table 1. $+p<0.05$; $*p<0.01$.

following repetitive irritation with a subclinical irritant. In his hypothesis repetitive subclinical irritation leads to a cumulative response if only the time interval between each irritation is short enough to prevent a complete recompensation of skin functions. Malten proposed a constant rate of skin regeneration. In contrary to his hypothesis, we were not able to confirm a pure cumulative response of skin function parameters following repetitive irritation with a surfactant as the irritant. In our study, we were able to show that there is a recompensation mechanism of the skin initiated by repetitive subclinical irritation. Therefore, Malten's hypothesis of a constant rate of skin regeneration is to be dismissed as a consequence of our results. Klein et al. [9] observed a reimprovement of barrier function after more than 14 days despite the continuation of repetitive irritation by dish-washing. Their observation was evaluated by TEWL measurements only. In our study, TEWL values increased steadily until day 5 and remained in a steady state thereafter until day 14. Comparing the TEWL results with the results of the other bioengineering methods used, there is obviously a delay of barrier function deterioration as well as a delay in barrier regeneration in comparison to skin hydration, skin blood flow and pH response following repetitive irritation. In conclusion, our study confirms the existence of a training effect following repetitive subclinical surfactant irritation of the skin. Regeneration of skin pH and skin hydration is observed first, followed by skin blood flow and finally by barrier function. Nevertheless, it remains an open question for future studies how prolongation (i.e. over more than 14 days) or intensification of irritation influence recompensation mechanisms.

Conclusions

Repetitive washing leads to deterioration of stratum corneum function, eventually progressing to the development of irritant contact dermatitis. In our previously published studies we repeatedly observed clinical improvement of the skin following maximum irritation despite the continuation of irriation. In this study we evaluated corneometry, TEWL, LD and pH values before and during repetitive irritation by a SLS solution. After the maximum of skin function deterioration between day 1 and day 5 of repetitive washings, skin function parameters slowly returned to a lower degree of deterioration within 14 days. In conclusion, we were able to show the existence of a training effect onto skin function parameters following repetitive washing.

References

1 Willis CM, Stephens CJM, Wilkinson JD: Experimental induced irritant contact dermatitis. Contact Dermatitis 1988;18:20–24.

2 Grunewald AM, Gloor M, Gehring W, Kleesz P: Damage to the skin by repetitive washings. Contact Dermatitis 1995;32:225–232.

3 Mosler U: Hautfeuchtigkeitsmessung – kein Problem mit dem Corneometer CM 420. Parf Kosm 1983;64:375–379.

4 Pinnagoda J, Tupker RA, Agner T, Serup J: Guidlines for transepidermal water loss measurement. Contact Dermatitis 1990;22:164–178.

5 Mahmoud G, Lachapelle JM: Evaluation of the protective value of an antisolvent gel by laser doppler flowmetry and histology. Contact Dermatitis 1985;13:14–19.

6 Post A, Gloor M, Gehring W: Über den Einfluss der Hautwaschung auf den Haut-pH-Wert. Dermatol Monatsschr 1992;178:216–222.

7 Tupker RA, Pinnagoda J, Coenraads PJ, Nater JP: The influence of repeated exposure to surfactants on the human skin as determined by transepidermal water loss and visual scoring. Contact Dermatitis 1989;20:108–114.

8 Malten KE: Thoughts on irritant contact dermatitis. Contact Dermatitis 1981;7:238–247.

9 Klein G, Grubauer G, Fritsch P: The influence of daily dish-washing with synthetic detergent on human skin. Br J Dermatol 1992;127:131–137.

Dr A.M. Grunewald, Am Wetterbach 52, D–76228 Karlsruhe (Germany)

Elsner P, Lachapelle JM, Wahlberg JE, Maibach HI (eds): Prevention of Contact Dermatitis. Curr Probl Dermatol. Basel, Karger, 1996, vol 25, pp 214–220

Moisturizers in the Prevention of Contact Dermatitis

Matti Hannuksela

South Karelia Central Hospital, Lappeenranta, Finland

Irritant dermatitis is the most important type of hand dermatitis. One of its most common causes is obviously the frequent use of detergents. Various creams and ointments, including ones called barrier creams, are used against both irritant and allergic contact dermatitis because of their preventive properties. Little is known, however, about the efficacy and the mode of action of such creams and ointments.

The Epidermal Barrier

The epidermal barrier is located in the horny layer. It has a 'brick and mortar' structure where the bricks are hydrophilic keratinocytes and the mortar consists of hydrophobic lipids. Cholesterol and its esters are said to account for 20–40% of the horny layer lipids, ceramides for 20–50%, fatty acids for 9–26% and others, such as squalene and triglycerides, for 3–17% (table 1). There are variations in the lipid content between the different parts of the body. The chain lengths of the fatty acids of the epidermal ceramides are usually 24–30 carbon atoms [4–6]. The chain length increases from the basal cells to the horny layer.

In addition to the lipids, the epidermis also contains other components influencing the water balance of the horny layer and the barrier function. Keratin fibres bind water, as does the natural moisturizing factor (NMF). NMF accounts for 15–20% of the weight of the stratum corneum. Its main components are amino acids (40%), inorganic salts (18.5%), pyrrolidone carboxylic acid (12%), lactates (12%) and urea (7%) [7].

Table 1. Composition of horny layer lipids according to the literature (percent of total, approximate values)

Component	Yardley and Summerly [1]	Lampe et al. [2]	Wertz and Downing [3]
Ceramides	49	20	39
Sterols	20	17	27
Sterol esters	0.7	6	10
Fatty acids	26	20	9
Other substances	2.6	30	13

In the traditional model of the lipid part of the epidermal barrier, the lipids make up bilamellar structures where the lipid units are randomly distributed. In 1994, Forslind [8] published 'the domain mosaic model' for the epidermal lipid barrier. In this model, lipids with very long chain lengths are segregated into domains in the crystalline/gel phase separated by grain borders populated by lipids with relatively short chain lengths in the liquid crystalline state.

Epidermal Barrier in Contact Dermatitis

The epidermal barrier is impaired in many skin conditions ranging from the xerotic skin of atopics to psoriasis. Eczematous dermatitis of the hands is a very common complaint among workers in wet work, especially those using detergents and solvents, and among workers handling foodstuffs. Detergents are thought to infiltrate primarily the fluid parts of the barrier, i.e. the grain borders in Forslind's model [8].

Detergents and solvents, and also plain water to some extent, dissolve lipids from the barrier. The transepidermal water loss increases and the skin turns rough, itchy and scaly.

In allergic contact dermatitis, the skin is inflamed and there is both intracellular and intercellular edema in the epidermis. In acute dermatitis, the horny layer is partly shed and tissue fluids are excreted fairly freely to the skin surface.

Moisturizers and Barrier Creams

Composition

Most moisturizers are oil-in-water creams with varying fat contents. Petrolatum, paraffins, tri- and diglycerides, lanolin or wool alcohols and waxes are the most common fats in them. Liposomes are popular in cosmetic creams, and they have recently been added to some o/w creams with or without active ingredients for the treatment of various dermatoses. Cetanol and stearol are used in creams both as emulsifiers and as fatty components. Creams and lotions may also contain glycerol, glycols, urea or some other humectants, i.e. substances with water-binding capacity. Silicones may be used in lotions and creams as water-resistant substances.

Water-in-oil creams, water-free ointments and waxes are also used as moisturizers. Silicones and polyethylene glycols are often added to them. Many patients find them cosmetically less acceptable than lotions and o/w creams.

Most barrier creams are nothing but usual o/w creams or ointments. Many of them contain silicones. Barrier creams usually resist water well. Some of them have been developed for special purposes, e.g. against solvents or cutting oils.

Effect of Ordinary Moisturizing Creams

Moisturizers are able to restore the water-holding capacity of the keratin layer at least to some extent. Petrolatum has been found to be the most effective moisturizer when the transepidermal water loss (TEWL) and dryness of the skin have been used as references [9, 10]. Other moisturizers are less effective than petrolatum in blocking TEWL, but they have better cosmetic acceptance among the consumers. Lodén et al. [11] examined the acceptance of 5 moisturizing creams. A cream with intermediate viscosity was considered more pleasant than creams with low or high viscosity. The grade of viscosity mostly depends on the amount of fats.

Hannuksela and Kinnunen [12] examined the effect of eight moisturizers on the prevention of irritant contact dermatitis in a wash test. The participants were medical students who washed the outer aspects of their upper arms with a dishwashing liquid for 1 min twice daily for 7 days. TEWL increased during the washing period by approximately 13 $g/m^2/h$ in the untreated arm, while the increase in the treated areas was only approximately 3 $g/m^2/h$. Itching and dermatitis appeared on the nontreated arm, while the treated areas remained objectively and subjectively free of symptoms and signs. Blood flow also increased significantly in the washed, nontreated arm, but did not change in the arm treated with moisturizers. During the second week, the dermatitis on the washed, nontreated arm disappeared and the laser Doppler values returned to normal. The TEWL values also decreased to a nearly normal level. The mean decrease was more pronounced when creams with a high fat content were used but, due to a notable interindividual variation, the differences between the results for the 8 moisturizers were not statistically significant. When the effect of a moisturizer was compared to no treatment after the 1-week washing period, the use of the moisturizer was found to enhance the healing process significantly.

Halkier-Sørensen and Thestrup-Pedersen [13] examined the efficacy of a moisturizer (Locobase®) among cleaners and kitchen assistants during everyday work. The study subjects used the moisturizer for 2 weeks and during a 1- or 2-week period they were not allowed to use any cream or lotion on their hands. The study was a cross-over study, and the study population was divided into two groups: those without a history of atopy and those with atopy. The atopics were allowed to shorten the period without moisturizers to 1 week. The study population used the moisturizer several times a day. It clearly prevented the development of dryness of the skin. The electrical capacitance (epidermal hydration) decreased significantly when the study subjects were not using the moisturizer but, unexpectedly, there was no increase in the TEWL rates or in skin temperature.

A water-in-oil emollient cream was shown to decrease significantly the number of cases of dermatitis among premature newborns in a neonatal intensive care unit [14]. In normal skin, a single application of a moisturizer did not cause long-lasting effects expressed as skin capacitance and conductance [15], whereas repeated applications of a moisturizer twice daily for 1 week produced a significant increase in the skin conductance for at least 1 week after cessation of treatment [16].

Canola oil and its sterol-enriched fraction were found to reduce SLS-induced irritation in human skin [17]. Neither fish oil nor borage oil influenced the degree of inflammation caused by SLS.

Both an oil-in-water cream and a water-in-oil cream, known as barrier creams, decreased the skin response to 10% SLS in large Finn Chamber tests. The former also decreased the effect of sodium hydroxide and lactic acid [18]. The authors pointed out the need for a reevaluation of the dogma that oil-in-water emulsions give a better barrier against lipophilic irritants and water-in-oil emulsions against hydrophilic irritants. The effects of barrier creams against industrial solvents and irritants, as well as against contact allergens are dealt with in the other chapters of this book.

Effect of Moisturizers with Active Ingredients

Urea-containing moisturizers have been a matter of controversion for more than two decades. Urea decreases reversibly the turnover of epidermal cells, which has been thought to impair the function of the epidermis [19–21].

A number of authors have reported an enhancing effect of urea on the permeability of various substances through the epidermis into the skin [19, 22–27] due rather to its direct effect on the keratin layer than to epidermal cell proliferation. Repeated applications of creams with 10% urea were shown to decrease the irritant effect of sodium laurylsulfate (SLS) on human skin, expressed both as the number of individuals reacting to SLS and as the change in the TEWL [17]. The mode of action of 10% urea could not be resolved in that particular study, because, contrary to 10% urea, three applications of a gel with 5% urea increased TEWL and skin capacitance. It is possible that a greater amount of urea alters the binding capacities of the stratum corneum, retarding the penetration of SLS. In another study, both a 3% urea cream and a 10% urea cream increased the hydration status of the skin and reduced scaling [28].

Triclosan has been claimed to be another substance that decreases the irritancy of SLS in human skin. Barkvoll and Rolla [29] made Finn Chamber® tests with SLS in 10 volunteers. SLS alone caused an irritant reaction in every person, while a mixture of SLS and triclosan caused no reactions. Pretreatment with triclosan showed only a slight decreasing effect whereas treatment after SLS exposure diminished the reactions to SLS significantly.

Clinical Significance of the Results of Experimental Studies

Only a few of the studies mentioned above were done on individuals with irritant dermatitis caused by their usual working or living conditions [13, 14] or by wash tests simulating exaggerated use of detergents [12]. Most investigators have utilized chamber tests. The results of various chamber tests have turned out to predict poorly the results of a wash test [30] or those of the repeated open application test (ROAT) with irritant substances [31].

New moisturizers will obviously be developed for the prevention of irritant contact dermatitis in the near future. Proper methods for inducing a standard irritant dermatitis will also be needed. In vivo experiments are the only way to evaluate the properties of moisturizers and barrier creams.

References

1 Yardley HJ, Summerly R: Lipid composition and metabolism in normal and diseased epidermis. Pharmacol Ther 1981;13:357–383.

2 Lampe MA, Burlingame AL, Whitney J, Williams ML, Brown BE, Roitman E, Elias PM: Human stratum corneum lipids: Characterization and regional variations. J Lipid Res 1983;24:120–130.

3 Wertz PW, Downing DT: Stratum corneum: Biological and biochemical considerations; in Hadgraft J, Guy RH (eds): Transdermal Drug Delivery: Developmental Issues and Research Initiatives. New York, Marcel Dekker, 1989, pp 1–22.

4 Gray GM, White RJ: Glycosphingolipids and ceramides in human and pig epidermis. J Invest Dermatol 1978;70:336–341.

5 Gray GM, White RJ: Epidermal lipid liposomes: A novel non-phospholipid membrane system. Biochem Soc Trans 1979;7:1129–1131.

6 Long SA, Wertz PW, Strauss JS, Downing DT: Human stratum corneum lipids and desquamation. Arch Dermatol Res 1985;277:284–287.

7 Jokura Y, Ishikawa S, Yamasaki S, Imokawa G: Solid state 13C-NMR studies on elastic property of the stratum corneum. 17th Int IFSCC Congr Yokohama, October 13–16, 1992 vol 2, pp 712–735.

8 Forslind B: A domain mosaic model of the skin barrier. Acta Derm Venereol 1994;74:1–6.

9 Agner T: An experimental study of irritant effects of urea in different vehicles. Acta Derm Venereol 1992;(suppl 177):44–46.

10 Lodén M: The increase in skin hydration after application of emollients with different amounts of lipids. Acta Derm Venereol 1992;72:327–330.

11 Lodén M, Olsson H, Skare L, Axéll T: Instrumental and sensory evaluation of the frictional response of the skin following a single application of five moisturizing creams. J Soc Cosmet Chem 1992; 43:13–20.

12 Hannuksela A, Kinnunen T: Moisturizers prevent irritant dermatitis. Acta Derm Venereol 1992; 72:42–44.

13 Halkier-Sørensen L, Thestrup-Pedersen K: The efficacy of a moisturizer (Locobase) among cleaners and kitchen assistants during everyday exposure to water and detergents. Contact Dermatitis 1993; 29:266–271.

14 Lane AT, Drost SS: Effects of repeated application of emollient cream to premature neonates' skin. Pediatrics 1993;92:415–419.

15 Blichmann CW, Serup J, Winther A: Effects of single application of a moisturizer: Evaporation of emulsion water, skin surface temperature, electrical conductance, electrical capacitance, and skin surface (emulsion) lipids. Acta Derm Venereol 1989;69:327–330.

16 Serup J, Winther A, Blichmann CW: Effects of repeated application of a moisturizer. Acta Derm Venereol 1989;69:457–459.

17 Lodén M: Biophysical properties of dry atopic and normal skin with special reference to effects of skin care products. Acta Derm Venereol 1995;(suppl 192):1–48.

18 Frosch PJ, Kurte A: Efficacy of skin barrier creams. IV. The repetitive irritation test (RIT) with a set of 4 standard irritants. Contact Dermatitis 1994;31:161–168.

19 Hellgren L, Larsson K: On the effect of urea on human epidermis. Dermatologica 1974;149:289–293.

20 Wohlrab W, Böhm W: Epidermisreaktion nach Langzeitenwirkung von Harnstoff. Dermatologica 1975;151:149–157.

21 Wohlrab W, Schiemann S: Untersuchungen zum Mechanismus der Harnstoffwirkung auf die Haut. Arch Dermatol Res 1976;255:23–30.

22 Allenby AC, Creasey NH, Edington AG, Fletcher JA, Schock C: Mechanisms of action of accelerants on skin penetration. Br J Dermatol 1969;81(suppl 4):47–55.

23 Feldman RJ, Maibach HI: Percutaneous penetration of hydrocortisone with urea. Arch Dermatol 1974;109:58–59.

24 Wohlrab W: The influence of urea on the penetration kinetics of topically applied corticosteroids. Acta Derm Venereol 1984;64:233–238.

25 Wohlrab W: The influence of urea on the penetration kinetics of vitamin-A-acid into human skin. Z Hautkr 1990;65:803–805.
26 Beastall J, Guy RH, Hadgraft J, Wilding I: The influence of urea on percutaneous absorption. Pharm Res 1986;3:294–297.
27 Kim CK, Kim J-J, Chi S-C, Shim C-K: Effect of fatty acids and urea on the penetration of ketoprofen through rat skin. Int J Pharm 1993;99:109–118.
28 Serup J: A double-blind comparison of two creams containing urea as the active ingredient: Assessment of efficacy and side-effects by non-invasive techniques and a clinical scoring scheme. Acta Derm Venereol 1992;(suppl 177):34–38.
29 Barkvoll P, Rolla G: Triclosan protects the skin against dermatitis caused by sodium lauryl sulphate exposure. J Clin Periodontol 1994;21:717–719.
30 Hannuksela A, Hannuksela M: Irritant effects of a detergent in wash and chamber tests. Contact Dermatitis 1995;32:163–166.
31 Hannuksela A, Hannuksela M: Irritant effects of a detergent in wash, chamber and repeated open application tests. Contact Dermatitis 1996;34:134–137.

Matti Hannuksela, MD, PhD, South Karelia Central Hospital, Valto Käkelän katu 4 A, FIN–53130 Lappeenranta (Finland)

Author Index

Subject Index